Musculoskeletal Medicine

D1197064

Series Editors

Grant Cooper, M.D.
Princeton Spine and Joint Center, Princeton, New Jersey, USA

Joseph E. Herrera, D.O.
Mount Sinai Medical Center, New York, NY, USA

For further volumes:
http://www.springer.com/series/7656

Ana Bracilović, M.D.

Essential Dance Medicine

Foreword by Donald J. Rose, M.D.

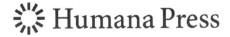 Humana Press

Ana Bracilović, M.D.
Princeton Spine and Joint Center
601 Ewing St., Suite A-1
Princeton, NJ 08540
USA
bracilov@gmail.com

ISBN 978-1-934115-67-1   e-ISBN 978-1-59745-546-6
DOI 10.1007/978-1-59745-546-6

Library of Congress Control Number: 2009921122

springer.com

For Lavko and Mila

Foreword

Dancers are unique, combining artistry and tremendous athletic skills. As a result, many of the musculoskeletal injuries sustained by dancers are unique. Recognition and subsequent management of these injuries therefore requires a special set of clinical skills, often different from those used to treat other athletic populations.

There have been great improvements in the recent past in the diagnosis and management of musculoskeletal injuries of dancers, which have taken advantage of recent advances in radiology (e.g., magnetic resonance imaging), surgery (e.g., arthroscopic techniques), and rehabilitation.

Doctor Bracilovic provides an up-to-date insight for all levels of healthcare practitioners into the recognition, background, and management of many of the common musculoskeletal injuries sustained by dancers. This is achieved in an easily digestible form, as a typical case presentation, diagnosis, scientific background and management of the injury, grouped by anatomic site. She approaches the text through her unique perspective as a dancer, an engineer, a researcher, and a physician specializing in physical medicine and rehabilitation.

It should also be mentioned that this text is not intended to be an all-inclusive compendium of the musculoskeletal evaluation and management of the injured dancer. Such knowledge can only be achieved by healthcare practitioners combining all available valid knowledge with their own experience in the management of dancers, recognizing their often unique psychological needs, and sharing their expertise and experience with others interested in benefiting this often underserved patient population. It is hoped that this text provides a valuable reference and stimulus toward this end.

Director, Harkness Center for Dance Injuries   Donald J. Rose, M.D.
NYU Hospital for Joint Diseases
Clinical Associate Professor
New York University School of Medicine

Preface

When I was 8 years old, I accompanied my father to karate classes. I liked the sensei and enjoyed memorizing the katas. Within a few months, I earned my yellow belt. Advancing in karate meant learning the "martial" part of martial arts and more advanced fighting maneuvers. When my mother came to class one day and watched me kick, punch, and get hurled to the ground, she feared I would get hurt. Once a serious student of ballet with great love for the art, she offered to enroll me in ballet classes. Ballet was a magical world of graceful, safe, and elegant movements accompanied by classical music that I had been playing on the piano since I was 5. I became smitten with dancing and began performing in recitals and competitions.

In high school, my goal was to become a brain surgeon, while my passion was dance. As an undergraduate, I remember spending hours in the bioengineering laboratory dissecting frogs' spinal cords and racing across campus to reach the studio in time for rehearsals. As artistic director of a university dance company, I loved performing, feeling the excitement of my fellow company members on stage and together experiencing the rush of sheer adrenalin and physical expression. Dance pieces were to me three-dimensional works of art, displaying beauty, athleticism, emotion, narration, and imagination.

In medical school, I was able to combine my fascination with the human body and its ability to display wide ranges of expression in choreography. Dance and medicine share a common base in human anatomy, kinesiology, and biomechanics. Dance demonstrates the body's incredible capacity for simultaneous strength and grace, agility and balance, stillness and fluidity. Medicine demonstrates its contrasts of health and pathology, ability and disability, autonomy and submission to disease.Dance displays the ultimate beauty of the body, medicine its nadir, and the potential to heal and return to optimal function.

In contrast to the apparent etherealness and ease of movement that ballet dance evokes, the physical demands of common ballet positions and the underlying principles of desired exaggerated lower extremity external rotation are entirely unnatural. Added to the requirements of dancing literally on the toes in pointe shoes, these positions and attributes are very difficult to attain. The effortlessness of ballet is an impressive illusion.

My intent in writing this book is to help medical professionals learn the presentations, differential diagnoses and available treatment options for common dance injuries. Too often, the career of a dancer is short lived and curtailed by poor injury prevention, improper dance technique, or nonspecific treatment. Even more frequently, if and when the dancer arrives at a doctor's office, the injury is in an advanced stage. It can often cost a professional dancer their career, and an amateur dancer their role in a performance. These tendencies have fostered a culture of inadequate education of all parties involved, from dancer, to teacher, to company director to medical professional. As members of a dance family, we have the responsibility and desire to make the careers of amateur and professional dancers healthy, long, and enjoyable. I hope this book helps accomplish that goal.

Ana Bracilović, MD
New York, 2008

Acknowledgments

To my husband Grant—my soul mate, inspiration, and MSA. ☼ My parents Ljubica and Dragomir—my earth, air, water, and sunshine. ☼ My brother Viktor—my role model of integrity and love. ☼ My parents-in-law Barbara and Joel—my support and good humor. ☼ Donald J. Rose MD—for his mentoring and enormous help with editing. ☼ Boni Rietveld MD, Elly Trepman MD, William Hamilton MD, Laurie Abramson, Lisa de Ravel, Risa Kaplowitz, and Mary Pat Robertson, PhD. ☼ The publishers of Humana Press – Springer for making this book possible. ☼ The beautiful members of Princeton Ballet School, Princeton Dance, and Theater Studio, my family, and colleagues who volunteered their time and creativity with this project: Jillian Brinberg, Christopher Costantini, Rachel Anne Costin, Jillian Davis, Lauren Elson MD, Allison, Emma, Robin and John Fleming, Francesca Forcella, Gretchen LaMotte, Aditi Menon MD, Drew Nelson, and Abigail Wohl.

Thank you.

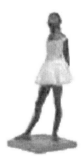

Contents

Introduction

From the 14th to 16th centuries, the Italian Renaissance fostered the art of Michelangelo, the political theories of Machiavelli, the architecture of Brunelleschi, and the art of ballet. Beginning in the 15th-century Italian court of the Medici family, classical ballet was brought by Catherine de Medici to France, where it further flourished during the 17th-century reign of Louis XIV.

Worldwide, ethnic and folk dance styles evolved with emphasis on dances of historical relevance. As choreographers introduced individual nuances and interpretations of traditional forms, classically trained dancers began exploring less restrictive technique, more expressive styles of free dance and theories of movement, from which early modern dance began. Neoclassical and contemporary ballet arose in the 20th century with faster tempos, more intricate jumps, oblique positions, flexed extremities, and more expansive use of stage space.

The classical ballet patterns described in this book characterize the seven commonly used training styles, including the Russian Vaganova method after Agrippina Vaganova, the Italian Cecchetti method after Enrico Cecchetti, the English Royal method after the Royal Academy of Dance, and the American Balanchine method after George Balanchine. The basic vocabulary of ballet positions and movements is similar across different training forms and is defined in this text to familiarize the reader. Specific figures depicting the most frequently used positions in classical ballet, modern and certain types of ethnic dance are illustrated.

As different types of dance have evolved, so have the injuries they keep. This text explains the underlying principles associated with correct ballet and modern dance movements in order to better understand the pathophysiology and mechanism of action for the injuries described. It also elucidates common errors and compensations dancers make in an effort to achieve correct positioning and technique.

As a field, dance medicine has continued to evolve over the past 20 years with increasing participation of former dancers, dance students, teachers, choreographers, and dance enthusiasts in the study of medicine, osteopathy, physical and occupational therapy, chiropractic, athletic training, acupuncture, and nutrition. Many factors contribute to the development of dance injuries, in addition to the physical demands of the art. Poor nutrition, eating disorders, stress and anxiety, inadequate dance floor surfaces, and footwear are all important factors contributing to the health of a dancer. Furthermore, injuries are often underreported as many dancers tend to "work through" their pain.

This text describes different types of dance injuries according to body region, including an initial case report that depicts a typical patient, followed by the epidemiology and pathophysiology associated with each injury. The history, physical examination findings, imaging, and diagnostic evaluation follow. Treatment describes options available for degrees of injury, according to chronicity and stages of severity. Non-operative and operative management is discussed. Relevant studies are cited as often as possible to provide evidence behind the algorithms of treatment and to highlight applicable research. Classic texts are also referenced to provide more in-depth information. May the dance begin.

1
Foot Injuries

Case Report   A 14-year-old modern jazz dancer who frequently dances barefoot comes to your office complaining of pain along the plantar aspect of her first metatarsal on both of her feet, right greater than left as well as deviation of her big toes toward her other toes making her feet look "crooked." She also complains of flat feet and calluses along the medial aspects of both first metatarsals.

Diagnosis   Hallux valgus

Epidemiology   Most common osteoarthritic joint of the foot. Most common pathologic condition of the great toe.

Pathophysiology   With increased valgus stress as seen in certain repetitive modern dance and ballet sequences, the head of the first metatarsal gradually moves medially, off of the sesamoid bones. The sesamoid bones remain attached to the proximal phalanx, and move in conjunction with it. As the valgus position worsens, the hallux pronates and rotates, typically forming a callus at the plantar aspect of the interphalangeal joint. Hallux valgus describes the deviation laterally from midline of the hallux by more than 15 degrees. Bunions represent a bony and soft-tissue first MTP joint deformity.

Dancers typically present with hallux valgus and bunions at a younger age than the general population, often as a result of **repetitive pronation in the "turned out" or externally rotated positions required in ballet dance**. The bunion and hallux valgus result from incorrect posture and biomechanics while attempting to achieve the often unnatural "turned out" position. The dancer will attempt to reach an externally rotated position of both hips with both feet directed laterally away from midline as much as possible. **The total degree of turnout involves a combination of femoral neck anteversion, femoral torsion, knee alignment, tibial torsion, and foot alignment.**

From: *Musculoskeletal Medicine*: *Essential Dance Medicine*
By A. Bracilović, DOI 10.1007/978-1-59745-546-6_1,
© Humana Press, a part of Springer Science+Business Media, LLC 2009

The five basic positions of ballet demonstrate this degree of alignment (Figures 1-1). Ideal turnout in ballet would involve 180 degree external rotation through the hip joints with alignment of the patellae over the second toes while maintaining elevation of the medial longitudinal arch. A straight plumb line would pass through the hip joint, bisect the patella, and fall over the second toe without hyperlordosis of the lumbar spine or pronation of the feet. Very few people possess this degree of "ideal" or "perfect" turnout. Humans are typically not built this way. Normally, the degree of femoral anteversion determining the amount of external rotation at the hip is 10 degrees. Femoral anteversion is measured by the angle formed by the plane of the femoral neck at the hip in relation to the plane of the femoral condyles at the knee.

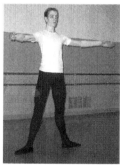

FIGURE 1-1. (**A**) Ideal turnout alignment.

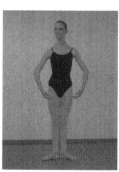

FIGURE 1-1. (**B**) First position.

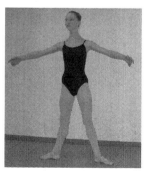

FIGURE 1-1. (**C**) Second position.

FIGURE 1-1. (**D**) Third position.

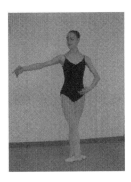

FIGURE 1-1. (**E**) Fourth position.

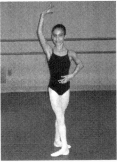

FIGURE 1-1. (**F**) Fifth position.

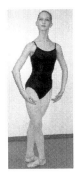

Dancers who do not have a significant degree of external rotation at the hips tend to compensate by trying to force external rotation at the knees, ankles, and feet with abnormal "wrenching" of the joints. Forcing external rotation at the hips increases femoral torsion. Forcing external rotation at the knees increases tibial torsion as the tibia rotates externally relative to the femur. Forcing external rotation at the hips and knees increases pronation of the foot at the subtalar joint in order to maintain neutral foot position. Bunions gradually form as a result of repetitive torquing of the feet in a turned out position with accompanying increased pronation.

History   Dancers typically present with gradual onset of foot pain over the ball of the foot and/or over the medial aspect of the first metatarsal head. Often, the bunions develop well before pain becomes a significant factor. When bunions do become painful, the pain is usually worse with weight bearing, jumping and at the end of rehearsals and/or classes. The pain is exacerbated with increased pressure over the tender area, which may include even direct palpation when the pain is severe.

PE   First, assess the range of motion of the MTP joint in the hallux valgus position as well as the normal anatomic position of the joint with passive correction. Also, note whether there is decreased range of motion when the hallux is placed in the correct position and whether there is hypermobility of the first metatarsal-cuneiform joint. Assess for degree of pronation of the hallux and presence of ligamentous laxity, which may be seen in young dancers. Pain may be elicited with the toe-off position during gait and tenderness may be present over the medial aspect of the MTP joint.

It is essential that the dancer be examined for alignment in the basic technical dance positions at the hip, knee, and ankle joints. Often, hallux valgus and bunions are manifestations of faulty underlying technique and biomechanics that a young dancer is unaware of when trying to reach the aesthetic appearance of the dance positions. It is also important to examine the dancer's technique in jumping, *plié*, and *relevé* and to assess any limitations in mobility.

Imaging/Diagnostic Evaluation   AP, lateral, lateral oblique, and sesamoid axial radiographs should be obtained in weight-bearing positions. The bunion may be best visualized on a lateral oblique view because of its location on the dorsomedial aspect of the metatarsal head.

Treatment   Patients with symptomatic hallux valgus should be identified early to potentially obtain the most benefit from conservative treatment. Patients with no evidence of degenerative joint disease of the MTP joint may find pain relief with a wide toe box. A stiff sole shoe, functional orthotics, and a toe spacer between the first and second toes can help with proper alignment and prevent progression of the injury. Lamb's wool placed around the tender area may alleviate the pain. The importance of **changing pointe shoes approximately every 6–8 months in young, growing dancers** and otherwise at least once a year should be emphasized. Additional modifications that may help reestablish normal alignment and biomechanics include insertion of a metatarsal pad underneath the second metatarsal to reduce excess load, adding to the height of the heel cup for increased control, and making a wider medial arch for a pronated or flat foot.

Surgery is to be considered only as a last resort and if the individual is unable to return to dance, as subsequent stiffness of the MTP joint may occur, precluding dancer's full range of motion. **Never operate on a dancer's bunion. An injury (if inevitable) should curtail the dancer's career and never the surgery.**

Case Report   A 60-year-old retired prima ballerina presents to your office complaining of burning pain in both of her great toes. The pain started gradually over the past year, worse with walking in high heels, and standing for long periods of time. She also complains of stiffness and decreased motion of both of her great toes.

Diagnosis   Hallux rigidus

Epidemiology   Most common osteoarthritic joint of the foot. Second most common pathologic condition of the great toe. Incidence of 1 in 40 individuals over the age of 50 [1]. Female to male ratio is 2:1.

Pathophysiology   Hallux rigidus typically arises in dancers who have decreased mobility in the first MTP joint. To achieve a full *demi pointe* position, the MTP joint reaches beyond 90 degrees of dorsiflexion. Dancers who either naturally lack this mobility or cannot gradually achieve it typically force the *demi pointe* position and subsequently jam the bones in the joint, causing impingement. Repeated forced dorsiflexion of the MTP joint in the *demi pointe* position as well as plantarflexion in the *en pointe* position can result in the formation of bone spurs, leading to even further reduced motion in the joint, accompanied by inflammation and worsening pain. Excessive pronation at the hallux in an attempt to force turnout of the feet can also add to the degenerative process.

History   The patient often presents with gradual onset of pain and decreased AROM around the hallux, worse with toe-off while walking, wearing high heels and standing. The pain is relieved with rest, associated with burning pain and/or paresthesias.

PE   On observation of gait, the patient will typically walk on the lateral border of the foot in a supinated position to avoid pressure on the painful area. Tenderness is typically elicited over the **dorsal** aspect of the hallux. On examination of the foot, decreased AROM of the hallux at the first MTP joint is observed, especially in dorsiflexion along with decreased PROM in dorsiflexion and often adequate ROM in plantarflexion. Normally, the hallux should have approximately 45 degrees of plantarflexion and 70 degrees of dorsiflexion.

The patient will typically **sickle** the foot in response to their lack of mobility, by inverting the foot at the ankle joint while rising in *relevé* to the *demi pointe* position. This relieves pressure off the first metatarsal and reduces the amount of impingement in the first MTP joint, however, increases the risk of ankle sprains and peroneal tendonitis in the long term and is neither technically nor aesthetically acceptable as a dance position (Figures 1-2).

Instead of sickling, the patient should be taught how to correctly achieve and maintain the *demi pointe* position. This is an anatomically safe and technically correct position that requires diligent practice to obtain. To avoid further injury and maintain correct alignment, it is imperative that the patient be instructed on this proper technique.

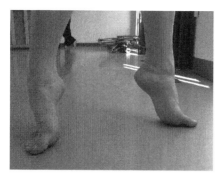

FIGURE 1-2. (**A**) Sickling rising in *relevé* to *demi-pointe*.

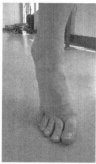

FIGURE 1-2. (**B**) Sickling anterior view.

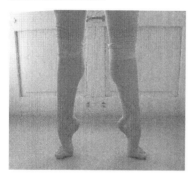

FIGURE 1-2. (**C**) Sickling corrected.

Imaging/Diagnostic Evaluation   AP, oblique, and lateral weight bearing radiographs typically show non-uniform joint space narrowing, widening and/ or flattening of the first metatarsal head and the base of the proximal phalanx. As the degenerative nature of the disease progresses, subchondral sclerosis or cysts may be seen, as well as sesamoid hypertrophy and osteophytes.

Treatment   In the acute phase, **PRICE** is recommended along with stretching of the foot in a pain-free range and non-weight bearing position (Figure 1-3) [2]. Physical therapy exercises should focus on stretching the hallux and sole of the foot within the patient's pain-free range of motion. Taping the hallux in a slightly plantarflexed position to avoid full *demi*

FIGURE 1-3. Stretching hallux.

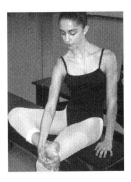

pointe can help restrict the painful extremes of motion. A molded stiff insert with a rigid bar or rocker bottom shoe may also be helpful.

Surgery is typically reserved for cases in which all attempts at non-operative management have failed. Specific procedures depend on the extent of deformity. Mild to moderate deformity typically is repaired with an uncomplicated cheilectomy. This procedure involves excision of dorsal and lateral osteophytes as well as the dorsal third of the metatarsal head. **For dancers, it is especially important to initiate passive and active range of motion exercises soon after surgery to restore adequate mobility of the joint.**

According to a study by Mulier et al. in 1999, excision of the osteophyte alone typically does not result in long-term pain relief [3]. Results from surgery and the ability to return to dance are variable and therefore operative management should be restricted only to those dancers who are unable to dance as a result of their injury.

Arthrodesis involves fusion of the first metatarsophalangeal joint and is reserved for cases in which cheilectomy has failed or where degeneration of the bone is severe. This procedure is restricted for dancers who have completed their dance career.

Case Report   A 19-year-old female ballet dancer presents to your office complaining of significant foot pain after rehearsing a pointe combination and abruptly rolling over onto the lateral border of her foot from *demi pointe*(Figures 1-4 and 1-5). She states that her foot buckled and she experienced immediate pain, swelling, and difficulty ambulating.

Diagnosis   Acute fracture of fifth metatarsal distal shaft, commonly known as "dancer's fracture"

Epidemiology   Most common acute fracture in ballet dancers.

Pathophysiology   A dancer's fracture usually occurs via an indirect mechanism, involving **twisting of the forefoot in a fixed position**. This can occur either as a result of rolling over and falling from the *demi pointe* position (on the ball of the foot with the ankle fully plantar flexed) (Figure 1-6) or from landing incorrectly onto an inverted and dorsiflexed foot. This results in a spiral, oblique fracture that originates distally and laterally and progresses proximally and medially. The fracture can often be displaced and occasionally comminuted. Peroneal weakness and/or a history of ankle instability can also predispose a dancer to this type of injury.

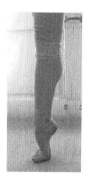

FIGURE 1-4. *Demi pointe* position.

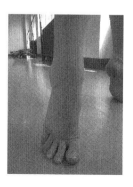

FIGURE   1-5. *Demi   pointe*   proper alignment.

FIGURE 1-6. Acute fifth metatarsal fracture mechanism of injury.

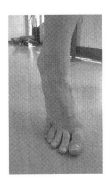

History   In dancers, this fracture most often occurs either during a performance or rehearsal and the patient will seek medical attention within 24 hours of injury. The patient will typically report pain and swelling over the lateral forefoot as a result of losing balance from the *demi pointe* position or landing incorrectly from a jump.

PE   Pain and bony point tenderness are elicited over the **lateral**aspect of the forefoot and along the fifth metatarsal, however, can be more generalized and often associated with swelling, ecchymosis, decreased active range of motion and difficulty, weight bearing.

Imaging/Diagnostic Evaluation   AP, lateral, and oblique radiographs of the foot should be obtained. Assessment of sagittal displacement of a fracture is important for appropriate management. If there is suspicion of a fracture and radiographs are negative, a bone scan can yield more information. It is more sensitive than plain radiographs, however, not specific. CT scan is helpful to determine intra-articular extension if the fracture is comminuted.

Treatment   Dancer's fractures are common injuries that can usually be treated **non-operatively**. Initially, protection, relative rest, ice to the injured area, compression to help prevent or reduce swelling, and elevation of the foot above the level of the heart (**PRICE**) form the mainstay of treatment. For dancers, rest and time off from rehearsals and/or performing are difficult doctors' orders to hear; however, the importance of preventing further injury to the already damaged area should be emphasized.

Initial rest and limitation of AROM to less than 10 degrees of angulation in any plane are usually recommended [4]. If the fracture is minimally displaced or **non-displaced**, a hard sole shoe or removable walker boot can initially be worn, with progression to full weight bearing in a hard sole shoe over 3–4 weeks. If the area of the fracture site is associated with significant swelling in the dancer, ankle range of motion is encouraged. Do not immobilize the dancer's ankle joint. If the fracture is **mild-moderately displaced** (3–5 mm), a short leg walker with weight bearing for 6–8 weeks is recommended. If the fracture is **grossly displaced** (> 5 mm) and/or significantly angulated, consider possible surgical reduction and internal fixation. **Surgical intervention is rare.** Closed reduction and percutaneous fixation may be necessary only when adequate reduction cannot be obtained, followed by gradual return to full weight bearing over 4–6 weeks.

O'Malley et al. in 1996 found that dancers with displaced fractures took longer to return to performance, with an average of 23 weeks, however did not find a correlation between the amount of displacement and final outcome, including residual pain or return to performance. Further, they reported a high rate of union and minimal long-term morbidity [5].

Rehabilitation following PRICE and any cast immobilization should include a full course of physical therapy for complete recovery and return to class and/or performance. Initially, the acute phase of physical therapy should include a training program with non-weight bearing activity, i.e. stationary biking or swimming. Following surgery, manipulation may be an option to restore AROM after a prolonged period of immobilization. The recovery phase of therapy focuses on PROM and AROM exercises, followed by stretching, strengthening, balance exercises, and restoration of proprioception.

Case Report A 21-year-old modern dancer collides with another dancer while balancing barefoot on *demi pointe*. She falls to the ground and experiences immediate pain and swelling over the lateral aspect of her left foot.

Diagnosis   Acute fracture of fifth metatarsal base: avulsion fracture

Epidemiology Most common fracture of base of fifth metatarsal.

Pathophysiology An acute fifth metatarsal base fracture is more specifically defined as a fracture occurring in the first of three previously classified fracture zones of the proximal fifth metatarsal [6]. Acute avulsion fractures typically occur in the first zone, which includes the insertion of the peroneus brevis tendon, the metatarsocuboid articulation, and the lateral plantar aponeurosis. Most often, the avulsion fracture is **extra-articular** and may extend intra-articularly. The avulsion fracture occurs through the tuberosity of the proximal metatarsal, perpendicular to the long axis and within the most proximal centimeter of the metatarsal. Similar to acute fifth metatarsal shaft fractures, acute fifth metatarsal base fractures occur most commonly via an indirect mechanism, involving **acute inversion of the foot**.

History The dancer will usually report an acute injury after forced inversion while on *demi pointe*, with the foot and ankle plantarflexed. It is often associated with acute onset of pain at the base of the fifth metatarsal.

PE Pain and bony point tenderness are elicited over the lateral aspect of the foot, worse with weight bearing. There is often focal tenderness to palpation over the proximal fifth metatarsal. The distal fibula and lateral ligamentous structures should also be examined to rule out any associated fracture and/or sprain, respectively.

Imaging/Diagnostic Evaluation AP, lateral, and oblique radiographs should be obtained to assess fracture location, possible displacement, intra-articular involvement and to distinguish acute avulsion and chronic stress fractures from Jones fractures.

Treatment Treatment is primarily symptomatic, for both non-displaced intra-articular and displaced fractures. Non-operative treatment following **PRICE** typically includes a hard sole shoe followed by a walker boot or short-leg walking cast for comfort for 4–6 weeks, with weight bearing as tolerated. A stirrup ankle brace may be helpful to limit the pull of the peroneus brevis on the metatarsal. Fractures typically heal by 6–8 weeks.

Operative treatment is rarely indicated for significantly large fractures that extend into the metatarsocuboid joint, involve greater than 30% of the articular surface or for symptomatic non-union. Typically, the small fragment is excised, followed by ORIF, closed reduction, and Kirschner wire fixation or tension band wiring.

Avulsion fractures typically heal with symptomatic care and progressive weight bearing and have a **good prognosis** for return to class and performance. Poor prognosis may be associated with posttraumatic arthritis.

Case Report   A 24-year-old professional dancer presents to your office complaining of pain over the lateral side of her foot with difficulty bearing weight for the past 2 days. She has been actively rehearsing an African dance piece that involves many jumps, leaps, and pivot turns on bare feet. She first felt the pain after an abrupt pivot turn while on *demi pointe.*

Diagnosis   Acute fracture of fifth metatarsal base: Jones fracture

Epidemiology   Occurs more frequently in ballet dancers and gymnasts [7]. Higher rate of delayed union and non-union.

Pathophysiology   True Jones fractures occur acutely at the metaphyseal--diaphyseal junction proximal to the metatarsocuboidal joint, classified previously as a Zone 2 injury by Dameron [3]. They are located slightly more distally than the aforementioned tuberosity avulsion fractures and are typically found 1–1.5 cm from the proximal metatarsal origin. This type of fracture tends to occur when the ankle is in a plantarflexed position and a large adduction force is applied to the forefoot, overloading the plantar aspect of the fifth metatarsal head. This in turn causes a significant bending stress with fracture of the bone occurring at the junction of the metaphysis and proximal diaphysis.

History   Many patients with true Jones fractures do not recall history of symptoms prior to the injury. Most commonly, the mechanism of injury is via **adduction** of the fifth metatarsal via a laterally directed force on the forefoot, with the foot in a **plantarflexed** position and the metatarsophalangeal joint **hyperextended**. Dance movements involving **abrupt pivoting** and change of direction on *demi pointe* mimic this mechanism of injury.

PE   Pain and tenderness are elicited over the fifth metatarsal base or proximal shaft. It is also important to examine the distal fibula, which may infrequently reveal an associated fracture.

Imaging/Diagnostic Evaluation   AP, lateral, and oblique radiographs should be obtained to assess fracture location, possible displacement, intra-articular involvement and to distinguish acute avulsion and chronic stress fractures from Jones fractures.

Treatment   Non-displaced Jones fractures can be treated in a non-weight bearing cast for 8–12 weeks in amateur or recreational performers; however, elite and professional dancers may opt for early operative intervention to avoid prolonged immobilization and the associated loss of strength and flexibility. Non-operative treatment is usually reserved for less than 3 month old, **minimally displaced** fractures without evidence of non-union on radiograph.

Displaced Jones fractures typically are treated with ORIF with intramedullary screw, followed by a non-weight bearing splint for one week, with progression to weight bearing using a walker boot for 2–3 weeks [8, 9].

Studies have reported that radiographic union typically occurs between 6 and 10 weeks and that return to full activity prior to complete radiographic union is predictive of failure. Since the diaphyseal–metaphyseal junction is a vascular watershed area, acute fractures are prone to delayed union or non-union. Dancers are generally recommended safe return to activity at about 10–12 weeks following the injury as risk of refracture is high. An adequate period of immobilization, shoe modification, functional bracing, orthoses, and additional imaging are recommended to reduce the incidence of refracture [10].

Case Report   A 19-year-old ballet dancer with history of anorexia nervosa comes to your office complaining of pain on the outside of her left foot for the past 3 weeks. She does not remember exactly when the pain started, but states that it has not improved and is now interfering with classes, rehearsals, and occasionally wakes her up at night.

Diagnosis   Stress fracture of fifth metatarsal base

Epidemiology   Higher frequency in modern dancers, gymnasts and with high impact aerobic activities.

Pathophysiology   Stress fractures of the fifth metatarsal base can occur as a result of excessive, repetitive, submaximal loading onto a bone. Anatomic causes include insufficient muscular, ligamentous, and/or tendinous support, improper biomechanical alignment and a suboptimal vascular supply. The mechanism of injury for a fifth metatarsal base fracture in a dancer typically occurs from **repetitive adduction** forces such as pivoting with the ankle plantarflexed as in most types of turns on one leg in *relevé*.

It has been reported that women have a greater disposition to stress fractures than men, and in particular dancers who exhibit the **female athlete triad** are at a higher risk for stress fractures and premature osteoporotic fractures. The female athlete triad consists of disordered eating, amenorrhea, and osteoporosis. Nutritional risk factors include inadequate calcium intake and hormonal factors include low circulating levels of estrogen in females associated with increased bone mineral density loss. Both oligomenorrheic and amenorrheic dancers have been shown in studies to have higher risk of bone loss, predisposing them to stress fractures [11].

History   In contrast to acute fractures, stress fractures are usually not associated with a traumatic history, rather by **insidious onset** of progressively worsening pain, localized to the bone and/or surrounding area involved. The patient may or may not report dance activity immediately prior to the pain, but as the pain progresses, it will occur more frequently during and following dance activity, then may interfere with activities of daily living and with sleeping at night. It typically improves with rest and is worse with ambulation, which is when the dancer typically takes note of it.

PE   Pain is elicited over the lateral aspect of the foot; however, may be difficult to localize. There may be associated edema and ecchymosis. It is also important to evaluate for ankle instability, limitation in subtalar joint motion, and presence of hindfoot varus, all of which can increase stress on the ankle and the fifth metatarsal [12].

Imaging/Diagnostic Evaluation   Anteroposterior, lateral, and oblique x-rays of the foot should be obtained. Initially, radiographs of stress fractures may be negative despite evident clinical symptoms, typically from 2 to 12 weeks following the injury. If there is suspicion of a fracture and x-rays are negative, serial radiographs, a bone scan, or MRI can be obtained.

Approximately 50% of stress fractures do not become evident on radiographs. Stress fracture findings on radiograph can include [2]:

1. Longitudinal cortical hypertrophy or lateral margin callus
2. Radiolucent widened fracture line
3. Medullary canal narrowing
4. Periosteal reaction

A convenient classification system of proximal diaphyseal fifth metatarsal fractures by Torg et al. arranges them according to healing potential [13]. Acute (**type I**) injuries are characterized by injury and onset of pain that are both acute. Radiographic findings include sharp fracture margins and minimal cortical hypertrophy and periosteal reaction. Delayed union (**type II**) fractures are characterized by a history of prior injury and persistent pain. Radiographic findings include mild fracture widening, new periosteal bone formation, and presence of intramedullary canal sclerosis. Non-union (**type III**) fractures are characterized by multiple prior injuries with recurrent symptoms. On radiograph, significant periosteal bone formation and complete intramedullary canal obliteration are seen.

Treatment   PRICE. For acute (**type I**) stress fractures, non-weight bearing ambulation is typically recommended for 6–8 weeks with progression to ambulation. For delayed union (**type II**) fractures in amateur dancers or those who do not require urgent return to high level activity, non-operative management with prolonged immobilization until union is achieved is typically adequate. Operative management is usually recommended for non-union (**type III**) and acute displaced fractures that have failed non-operative management as well as elite dancers with type II stress fractures who prefer surgical treatment and/or need to return to rehearsing or performing. Surgical intervention usually involves ORIF, closed reduction with intramedullary screw or Kirschner wire fixation, bone graft or tension band wiring. With closed treatment, the rate of non-union is 50%; therefore, the dancer may benefit from early intervention with ORIF.

Return to class, rehearsal, and/or performance can be introduced gradually with progressive increase in intensity and duration of activity. In general, the intensity and duration should not increase more than 10% from week to week. Rest intervals should be frequent, and pain-inducing activities should be avoided. If pain does recur, activity should be resumed at a lower level of difficulty and only when pain free.

Case Report A 26-year-old professional ballet dancer is rehearsing a variation *en pointe* and complains of persistent pain over the middle part of her foot worsening over the past few weeks. She does not remember an acute injury.

Diagnosis   Stress fracture of second metatarsal base

Epidemiology Common stress fracture in female ballet dancers.

Pathophysiology This type of fracture occurs most often with the ankle fully plantarflexed and the forefoot plantarflexed, as in the *en pointe* position in female ballet dancers. Normally, when the foot is flat on the ground, the ankle serves as an articulation between the foot and the leg, allowing each to perform as a separate lever. In the *en pointe* position, however, the foot is fully plantarflexed at the ankle and forms a single long lever arm with a large concentrated force at the second tarsometatarsal junction (Figure 1-7).

Lisfranc's joint is the site of articulation of the second metatarsal and three cuneiform bones. The base of this articulation is at the proximal middle cuneiform, with the adjacent medial and lateral cuneiform articulations securing the proximal second metatarsal head into a relatively inflexible socket. This unique anatomic configuration has three important characteristics:

1. It predisposes Lisfranc's joint to injury.
2. It significantly reduces the mobility of the second metatarsal joint in comparison with the other metatarsal joints.
3. It provides the locking mechanism for the tarsometatarsal complex.

Patients with a Grecian or Morton's foot, characterized by a hypermobile, short hallux and longer second toe (Figure 1-8), as well as those with increased passive external hip rotation greater than 60 degrees have been reported to have a higher incidence of second metatarsal stress fractures [14]. Poor nutrition and amenorrhea have also been cited as risk factors.

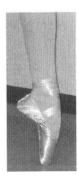

FIGURE 1-7. Foot fully plantarflexed *en pointe*.

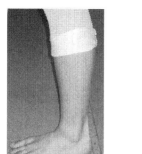

FIGURE 1-8. Grecian (Morton's) foot.

History   The patient is most often female, as the injury nearly exclusively occurs in ballet dancers in the *en pointe* position, performed only by female dancers. The dancer will typically complain of pain in the midfoot. It is important to diagnose this type of fracture early, as a delayed or missed diagnosis can allow the fracture to progress, resulting in non-union and subsequent operative intervention that could have been avoided.

PE   Tenderness is elicited with palpation over the joint with associated pain in passive abduction and pronation of the forefoot while holding the hindfoot fixed. There may be associated localized edema.

Imaging/Diagnostic Evaluation   Anterior–posterior, lateral, and oblique radiographs of the foot should be obtained. Conventional radiographs often will not reveal a stress fracture in the first 2 weeks following injury. Triple phase bone scan has good sensitivity but poor specificity and can demonstrate evidence of a stress fracture within 24–72 hours from the time of injury. MRI is more expensive but is quickly becoming the study of choice with sensitivity comparable to a bone scan but much improved specificity.

Treatment   PRICE. If diagnosed promptly, the fracture can be expected to heal with an initial period of immobilization in a post-operative, wooden soled shoe or short removable walker boot. If the fracture is associated with marked pain, swelling and/or minimal evidence of healing, this may be followed by a short-leg (below knee) walking cast for 6 weeks.

An orthopedic surgeon should be consulted for any second metatarsal fracture that does not demonstrate evidence of radiographic healing after 6 weeks of non-surgical treatment. The patient may gradually return to dance with slow increase in duration and intensity of activity. The rate of increase in dance activity should not exceed 10% per week. Activity should be limited to pain free range of motion and frequent rest periods included. Return to dance may be prolonged with this type of injury. Surgery is indicated only upon evidence of stress fracture non-union.

Case Report   A 30-year-old male modern dancer presents to your office complaining of pain in his left midfoot after being knocked over by a fellow modern dancer while pivoting sharply on his left foot. He notes that *relevé* and weight bearing on his left leg are difficult.

Diagnosis   Midfoot (Lisfranc's) sprain

Epidemiology   More commonly associated with Irish dancers, underdiagnosed midfoot injury [15].

Pathophysiology   Whereas the bases of the second through fifth metatarsals are connected by strong plantar transverse metatarsal ligaments, Lisfranc's ligament runs obliquely from the medial cuneiform to the second metatarsal base, providing stability to the first two toes. In dancers, proper pointe technique involves plantarflexion at the transverse tarsal or Chopart's joint (Figure 1-9). Mechanisms of injury include axial loading onto a foot that is plantarflexed at the transverse tarsal joint on *demi pointe* combined with either rotation or forced abduction of the forefoot. The dorsal ligament complex of the tarsometatarsal joint is compromised [16]. Often, dancers will force plantarflexion at the first and second metatarsal cuneiform joints, which can overstretch the surrounding ligaments, cause hypermobility of the joint, and ultimately result in instability.

History   The patient will typically present complaining of midfoot pain and swelling associated with decreased ability to bear weight or *relevé* on one leg. The pain is usually associated with a forceful twisting of the affected foot while on *demi pointe* with the ankle plantarflexed with either sharp pivoting or being knocked over by a fellow dancer. Alternatively, a female ballet dancer may report loss of balance while *en pointe* and turning, leading to an excessively plantarflexed position of the transverse talar joint.

PE   On exam, there is typically tenderness to palpation over the base of the first and second metatarsals. Rising in *relevé* on the affected leg in active plantarflexion will be difficult. Provocative testing will reveal pain with passive pronation with simultaneous abduction of the midfoot and forefoot.

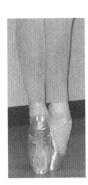

FIGURE 1-9. Plantarflexion at transverse tarsal (Chopart's) joint.

The midfoot may be swollen and ecchymotic. It is important to identify joint instability if present.

Imaging/Diagnostic Evaluation   AP, lateral, oblique, and bilateral weight bearing films of the foot should be obtained to rule out fracture and abnormal bony alignment. Radiographs will reveal the possible presence of a diastasis between the first and second metatarsal bases or associated avulsion fractures.

Treatment   Once diastasis, joint instability or associated avulsion fractures are ruled out, non-operative treatment can begin. **PRICE** is instituted in the acute phase. Initially, the foot is placed in a short leg walking boot or wooden shoe provided there is no evidence of either clinical or radiographic instability. This is followed by progressive weight bearing as tolerated. Depending on the patient and the degree of injury, stable sprains may take a minimum of 6–8 weeks to heal. Return to rehearsals and full dance activity may be prolonged, sometimes requiring 3–6 months of rehabilitation. If diastasis or joint instability is present, surgery may be indicated.

Case Report   A 30-year-old modern dancer and marathon runner presents to your office complaining of worsening pain over the dorsal aspect of her left midfoot over the past 2 months. The pain occasionally radiates down the inner arch of her foot. She previously had a radiograph that was normal.

Diagnosis   Tarsal navicular stress fracture

Epidemiology   Uncommon and often underdiagnosed injury in dancers, may account for approximately 29% of stress fractures in athletes [17]

Pathophysiology   The navicular bone contributes to normal gait as part of the medial longitudinal arch as well as the transverse tarsal (also known as the midtarsal or Chopart) joint. A stress fracture in this area can have multiple etiologies, most commonly arising from the repetitive load of jumping on a hard surface with improper biomechanics.

History   As this injury is uncommon and underdiagnosed in dancers, one should suspect a tarsal navicular stress fracture in a patient with unexplained midfoot pain. Often a history of frequent jumping can be elicited, although the pain is usually not associated with a single traumatic event and may have been present for weeks to months. The pain is typically worse with activity, better with rest, and can be associated with mild swelling over the dorsal midfoot. The patient can present with dorsomedial foot pain that is difficult to localize. The pain may radiate along the dorsum of midfoot, medial longitudinal arch, or first or second ray.

PE   The patient may have tenderness to palpation over the proximal dorsal aspect of the navicular bone or at the midmedial arch over the navicular bone. Passive eversion and active inversion may reproduce the pain as well as jumping with the foot inverted and the ankle plantarflexed.

Imaging/Diagnostic Evaluation   CT or MRI should be obtained to delineate treatment. Navicular stress fractures are typically not visible on plain radiographs. A negative radiograph does not rule out a navicular stress fracture. The lateral fragment of a navicular fracture may appear as a separate tarsal bone on an AP radiograph and overlooked if one does not carefully follow the continuity of the cortical bone. A technetium bone scan is sensitive but not specific for a navicular stress fracture and will show increased uptake at the navicular fracture site. CT is considered standard of care for diagnosis and MRI can be helpful for grading the stress fracture severity and guiding the course of treatment.

Treatment   Presence of a cortical defect typically requires immobilization in a non-weight bearing cast for 6–8 weeks to appropriately heal. **Complete or displaced** fractures typically require surgical intervention with a combination of screw fixation and bone grafting. Weight bearing activity may begin once there is no longer focal tenderness over the navicular bone. Physical therapy should initially focus on strengthening and ROM of exercises, as well as soft tissue mobilization. An orthotic with indwelling longitudinal and transverse arch supports can be helpful and decrease pressure on the affected area. **Pain free range of motion** should be emphasized with all activity.

Case Report   A 27-year-old Broadway musical dancer presents to your office complaining of pain underneath her right big toe for the past 8 weeks. She recently returned from a traveling tour where she was performing in character shoes in multiple venues. Many of the hardwood surfaces irritated her feet. When taking a break from performing, she spent a significant amount of time walking barefoot on the beach, which she states also exacerbated her pain.

Diagnosis   Sesamoiditis

Epidemiology   Injury to sesamoids common following inadequate *plié* upon landing from jumps.

Pathophysiology   The sesamoid bones, of which there are usually two, are unique in that they are not connected to any other bones in body. They lie within the medial and lateral heads of the flexor hallucis brevis (FHB) tendon, with contribution from the abductor and adductor hallucis tendons. With weight bearing, and most often when in *relevé*, the tibial sesamoid receives proportionally more weight than the fibular sesamoid and thus is injured more often. The tibial sesamoid bone is located medially and is usually longer and larger than the more lateral fibular sesamoid. In the push-off phase of the normal gait cycle, the sesamoids transmit forces up to three times body weight [18]. Inflammation and swelling surrounding the sesamoids and involving the FHB can occur as a result of trauma, stress fracture, infection, avascular necrosis, or systemic disease.

In dancers, predisposing factors are commonly errors in technique, which can range from hip to toe. These include sacroiliac joint dysfunction, incorrect landings from jumps, forced turnout from the feet causing overpronation and repetitive movement from flat to *demi pointe* or full *pointe*. Differences in foot and sesamoid anatomy may predispose a dancer to sesamoiditis. For example, an excessively thick or pointed sesamoid may result in callus formation around the area, whereas a cavus foot may result in excess weight bearing underneath the first metatarsal.

History   The patient will typically have pain with weight bearing and dorsiflexion of the great toe. Often, the patient will compensate for the pain on the plantar aspect of the first metatarsal by transferring weight to the lateral plantar aspect of the foot. This is most easily accomplished by a maneuver known as **sickling**, which is characterized by inversion of the foot at the ankle joint while the dancer rises in *relevé* to the *demi pointe* position (Figure 1-10). Compensation in this position puts excessive stress on the lateral ankle ligaments and lateral metatarsal bones, predisposing to increased risk of ankle sprain and fifth metatarsal fractures. It is neither a technically nor aesthetically acceptable dance position.

PE   Initial evaluation of gait is important to observe in a patient with sesamoiditis, although the acute painful area is in the foot. A tight hip

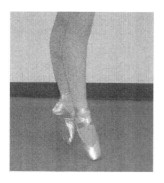

FIGURE 1-10. Right foot sickling *en pointe*.

capsule, sacroiliac joint dysfunction, and/or increased pronation of the feet all reflect abnormal underlying biomechanics that may be causing the patient to overload the sesamoid bones. Clinical exam will likely reveal tenderness to palpation and/or swelling over the medial sesamoid, more frequently than the lateral. Active resisted MTP flexion will often be painful, as well as passive, forced dorsiflexion of the hallux with one hand while palpating the plantar surface of the first MTP joint with the opposite thumb. However, if pain is not elicited, ask the patient to *relevé*, and assess for pain in this weight-bearing position.

Imaging/Diagnostic Evaluation   AP, lateral, oblique, and sesamoid view radiographs should be obtained to rule out sesamoid and/or stress fractures. If the fracture is not visualized on radiograph but there is high suspicion of a stress fracture, a nuclear bone scan or MRI can be helpful. An injection of lidocaine into the bursa beneath the sesamoids is diagnostic.

Treatment   The two main goals of treatment of sesamoiditis are to **minimize**weight bearing on the sesamoids and metatarsal joint flexion during ambulation. Initially, limit the patient's dance activity on *demi pointe* and educate the patient on realignment of appropriate biomechanics of the hip, sacroiliac joint, knee, ankle, and foot. Emphasize avoiding forced turnout and working within their natural range of motion. Rehabilitation of the patient with sesamoiditis should begin with *demi pointe* exercises on both feet, followed by *demi pointe* exercises on one foot, followed by jumps on both feet, then jumps onto one foot. It is also important to **emphasize stretching of both the flexor hallucis longus (FHL) and the FHB tendons**. Although the pathology may be localized to the FHB tendon, rehabilitation should include stretching of both tendons.

   It is usually appropriate to begin treatment with shoe modifications and extra-soft shoe inserts. A J-shaped pad or dancer's pad should be placed below the affected sesamoid to relieve pressure in that area. A full length steel shank and anterior rocker bottom are also recommended, and can be used for other conditions, including turf toe [19]. Taping of the toe in a

1. Foot Injuries   25

slightly plantarflexed position may also be helpful. The idea is to reduce dorsiflexion of the hallux and subsequently minimize the stress of weight bearing on the sesamoids. If the use of physical therapy, foot pads, inserts, and taping does not work, consider oral non-steroidal anti-inflammatory medications (NSAIDs) in the acute painful phase. Corticosteroid injections are **not** recommended.

Surgery should typically be regarded as a last resort as this may result in the dancer being unable to return to dance. Single sesamoidectomy in particular should be avoided, as this procedure can result in excessive stress placed on the remaining sesamoid bone [20]. Surgery is most often reserved for tibial sesamoid non-union, bipartite sesamoid, or for symptoms that have not resolved despite non-operative attempts greater than 6 months. The smaller sesamoid fragment is removed, followed by reattachment of the FHB tendon to the remaining sesamoid. Excising both sesamoids is typically avoided as it can lead to a "cock up" deformity. Excising only the tibial sesamoid can lead to hallux valgus and excising only the fibular sesamoid can lead to hallux varus.

Case Report   A 22-year-old male ballet dancer reports tenderness over the dorsal aspect of his left big toe that initially began about a year ago after accidentally forcing the toe abruptly into plantarflexion. The initial pain went away, but he has recently been noticing decreased range of motion in the joint when attempting multiple *pirouette*s and balancing on the left foot.

Diagnosis   First metatarsophalangeal (MTP) joint sprain, also known as "turf toe"

Epidemiology   Increased risk with foot pronation, flexible toe box, increased friction between dance shoe and dance surface [21].

Pathophysiology   The first metatarsal bears approximately one-third the body's weight via its two sesamoid bones beneath the metatarsal head and is thus essential for weight-bearing activities. Normally, the hallux supports 40–60% of our body weight while walking [22] with increased load during jumps in dance. It is also an interesting joint in that unlike a typical hinge joint the first MTP joint moves through multiple planes, including rolling and sliding, comparable to the range of motion of a shoulder or hip joint. The plantar complex forming the capsule of the first MTP joint is comprised of muscles, tendons, and ligaments as well as a strong fibrous structure called the plantar plate that loosely attaches to its origin at the metatarsal neck and more firmly attaches to the proximal phalanx. It combines with the flexor hallucis brevis tendons and the sesamoid bones for structural support.

The relevance of this anatomy is important when considering the mechanism of injury of first MTP joint sprains. When a dancer catches her first toe in a soft ballet shoe and forcefully hyperextends the first MTP joint, the plantar complex is stressed and can potentially tear at the weaker metarsal neck attachment or distal to the sesamoids. Also known as "turf toe" in athletes who play sports on grass or artificial "turf" surfaces, first metatarsophalangeal joint sprains are seen in ballet dancers wearing soft ballet shoes. While the soft flat shoe allows for easier and wider range of motion than the hard pointe shoe, significantly higher stresses occur across the forefoot in a soft shoe.

History   While occurring far less frequently than ankle sprains, it is important to suspect first MTP joint sprain as improper treatment can lead to persistent pain and loss of ROM. The patient will typically report having been positioned on *demi pointe* with the forefoot fixed on the ground and having **"caught" the shoe on the floor** on intended push-off, forcing the first metatarsophalangeal joint into further dorsiflexion.

PE   Localized tenderness to palpation over the plantar plate, dorsal capsule, sesamoids, and/or collateral ligaments may be noted, along with associated minimal to mild swelling and ecchymosis. The patient will typically have decreased AROM in dorsiflexion and plantarflexion but should be able to continue participating in dance activities. There may be associated instability or hypermobility that may reflect tear of the plantar plate, capsule, or associated ligaments. Instability is assessed with the dorsoplantar drawer test of the first MTP joint (Figures 1-11). Varus and valgus stress tests assess integrity of the collateral ligaments. **Grade I** injuries typically present with localized tenderness, minimal swelling, and no ecchymosis. **Grade II** injuries involve more diffuse tenderness, mild-moderate swelling, and ecchymosis. **Grade III** injuries are frequently associated with diffuse tenderness, swelling, and moderate to severe ecchymosis. The patient is unable to bear weight and has painful range of motion. Keep in mind clinical findings that may need surgical intervention, including decreased toe flexor strength, toe clawing or misalignment, and/or instability of the hallux or foot [23].

Imaging/Diagnostic Evaluation   AP weight-bearing, lateral, and sesamoid axial views should be obtained to rule out fractures, abnormal alignment, or diastasis. Contralateral views are often recommended to compare sesamoid-to-joint distance differences from normative values. Stress radiographs can reveal ligamentous instability. MRI is usually not needed; however, will be able to better define bony, joint, or soft tissue injury.

Treatment   Similar to lateral ankle sprains, first MTP joint sprains are typically divided into grades of injury according to severity. These have been previously characterized for "turf toe" injuries most commonly seen in football players, but can be applied to a similar mechanism of injury in ballet dancers.

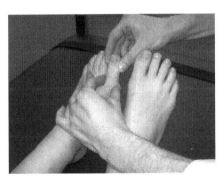

FIGURE 1-11. (**A**) Dorsoplantar drawer test first MTP joint.

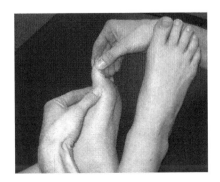

FIGURE 1-11. (**B**) Dorsoplantar drawer test first MTP joint sagittal view.

Protocols of therapy vary depending on the severity of injury. Acutely, however, **PRICE** is recommended for all grades of injury. **Grade I** injuries can then be treated with figure of 8 taping around the hallux to prevent excessive plantarflexion. The patient can typically return to dance within pain-free range of motion activity. In street shoes, the flexible insole should be replaced with a stiff steel or graphite footplate beneath the forefoot to avoid excess range of motion and subsequent loss of stability.

Grade II injuries require PRICE acutely, followed by immobilization in a hard sole shoe or removable walker boot for the first week with gradual return of first MTP range of motion. The patient can typically return to dance over the next 2–4 weeks. **Grade III** injuries require immobilization in a short leg cast with a toe spica in slight plantarflexion or removable walker boot to allow for soft tissue healing, followed by gradual ROM exercises 3–5 days following injury as tolerated by pain. Typically, the patient will require 2–6 weeks off from dance activities.

If non-operative treatment fails or if the sprain is associated with unstable ligamentous injuries, displaced intra-articular fractures or irreducible dislocations, surgery may be considered.

Criteria for return to dance should typically include pain free passive range of motion of the hallux in a range comparable to the contralateral (presumably normal) side. Remember to remind the patient that compensation with weight bearing on the lateral aspect of the foot is not an acceptable option if the patient continues to have pain as this can lead to associated injuries on the lateral aspect of foot. It is important to give this injury adequate time to heal as continued irritation can lead to osteophyte formation on the dorsal aspect of the MTP joint. Continued spurring can lead to decreased range of motion, persistent pain, and eventually hallux rigidus.

Case Report   A 16-year-old dancer who is the tallest student in her ballet class presents to you complaining of forefoot pain that is worse with *relevé* and improves with rest.

Diagnosis   Metatarsophalangeal synovitis

Epidemiology   Most often occurs between 12 and 20 years of age.

Pathophysiology   The normal range of motion in the first metatarsophalangeal joint is approximately 50–70 degrees of dorsiflexion and 30–50 degrees of plantarflexion. In dancers, achieving a full *relevé* from flat foot through *demi pointe* to full *pointe* position requires approximately 90–100 degrees of dorsiflexion. Given this often unnatural required range of motion of the joint, many young dancers will attempt to attain increased mobility with increased stress on the growing epiphysis. Repetitive excessive dorsiflexion and plantarflexion of the joint can occasionally lead to inflammation of the epiphysis and surrounding synovium, associated with pain and swelling. Metatarsophalangeal synovitis can also occur as a result of an acute trauma, where a microfracture occurs at the epiphyseal plate and interrupts its blood supply.

History   The patient will typically complain of pain in the forefoot at the level of the first metatarsal head, increased with standing, walking, and progressing through *relevé* to *demi pointe*. The pain usually subsides with rest. The patient will often avoid pressure on the anterior arch of the foot and place more pressure on the lateral aspect of the foot.

PE   On exam, the foot itself usually has no apparent superficial pathology. There may be tenderness to palpation over the dorsal or plantar surface of the first metatarsal head. Range of motion of the first phalanx should be normal, unless the patient presents after several weeks of symptoms. In this stage, there may be slight erythema and associated swelling of the forefoot. Range of motion of the first phalanx may be restricted and painful.

Imaging/Diagnostic Evaluation   AP and oblique radiographs should be obtained. When revealing, the radiograph can show changes in the metatarsal bone at the epiphysis including irregular contours and an indented, flattened articular surface.

Treatment   This condition tends to recur in adolescents, but typically resolves when the epiphyses fuse at maturity, at approximately 18–20 years of age. Initially, **PRICE** is the mainstay of treatment. Dance activity should be limited for 4–6 weeks until the patient's symptoms improve and gradually return to dance within pain-free range of motion. Consider NSAIDs in the acute stage to help relieve pain. **Premature closure of the physis may occur if the injury is not appropriately managed.**

Case Report   A 25-year-old female *corps de ballet* dancer presents to your office complaining of pain over the lateral aspect of her right foot that has gradually been worsening over the past year. She does not recall any trauma or specific injury to her foot. She has tried oral anti-inflammatories and physical therapy without significant relief of her symptoms.

Diagnosis   Cuboid subluxation

Epidemiology   Can occur acutely with ankle sprains [24].

Pathophysiology   Cuboid subluxation can occur acutely or develop as a chronic condition. Its existence as a condition has been disputed and is not universally accepted. It poses a controversial issue because the subluxation cannot be confirmed with imaging and no clinical symptoms exactly describe it. In male dancers, it can result from incorrect jump landing. Cuboid subluxation may also occur with lateral ankle sprains or as a result of repetitive transition from the flat foot position with the ankle dorsiflexed to full plantarflexion in the *en pointe* position. This process is seen in female ballet dancers. Repetitively rising from flat foot to *demi pointe* through to full *pointe* involves changing the direction of the applied force on the midfoot, leading to increased stress and decreased stability in this area. Typically, the medial aspect of the cuboid will sublux inferiorly with resultant superior displacement of the fourth metatarsal base and inferior displacement of the fourth metatarsal head.

History   If a patient presents with peroneal tendonitis, include cuboid pathology in the differential diagnosis as cuboid pathology can result in peroneal tendon dysfunction. The patient will typically complain of lateral midfoot pain that has persisted for some time and may be associated with weakness in toe-off. There may also be associated radiating pain to the fourth ray or plantar medial foot. He or she may report a prior ankle sprain that was resistant to conservative treatment.

PE   Tenderness is typically elicited with dorsally directed pressure over the plantar surface of the cuboid. Decreased active range of motion in the affected foot compared to the contralateral side can be seen. Range of motion is also reduced in passive pronation and supination. A gap may be felt at the base of the fourth metatarsal if the cuboid is significantly subluxed. The patient may have difficulty bearing weight, depending on the severity of injury.

Imaging/Diagnostic Evaluation   Radiographs may be obtained if this injury is associated with trauma. Minimal subluxation of the cuboid may be present even in asymptomatic patients. Imaging studies are usually unremarkable.

Treatment   Treatment is initially aimed at mobilization of the hindfoot and midfoot with adduction of the forefoot. Various techniques of cuboid manipulation have also been described previously, and most have been adapted to the cuboid "squeeze" described by Marshall and Hamilton [25]. This has been identified as a safer and more controlled maneuver that eliminates the high force transmitted to the talocrural joint from "whipping" the foot as seen in the cuboid "thrust" technique. In the cuboid squeeze, the ankle joint is held in slight plantarflexion with the plantar surface of the patient's foot in the examiner's hands. The midfoot is stabilized by placing both thumbs on the medial plantar surface of the cuboid and the fingers along the dorsolateral aspect of the foot. A direct dorsal force is applied to the medial aspect of the cuboid. The examiner may or may not feel a shift of the cuboid beneath the fingers. If the reduction is successful, the patient will typically have symptomatic relief.

Physical therapy should focus on strengthening the peroneal muscles and training the dancer in the flat foot position as well as *en pointe*. Stretching of the gastrocnemius and soleus muscles is also important, as well as emphasizing balance and proprioception retraining. Return to dance should be gradually introduced with exercises beginning at the barre followed by center work. Low dye arch taping and cuboid padding are also often used. The padding is usually ¼ inch thick and placed directly underneath the cuboid without extension to the fifth metatarsal.

Case Report   A 40-year-old female Broadway dancer presents complaining of a dull cramping sensation over the plantar aspect of the space in between the third and the fourth toes of her right foot. She frequently wears high heels and tight-fitting shoes in her role in the production of "Hairspray." She states she occasionally has some numbness and burning in the same area.

Diagnosis   Interdigital (Morton's) neuroma

Epidemiology   Most commonly affects females between 15 and 50 years old.

Pathophysiology   The interdigital nerves travel inferior to the intermetatarsal ligament and may be compressed or stretched at the level of the metatarsal heads. The term neuroma is actually a misnomer as this condition refers to entrapment of the plantar interdigital nerve as it passes under the transverse metatarsal ligament. In dancers, repetitive toe dorsiflexion and plantarflexion through *relevé*, *plié*, pivoting, and jumping may lead to demyelination and/or perineural fibrosis of the involved interdigital nerves. Dancers with tight gastrocnemius and soleus muscles as well as those who tend to pronate their feet may compensate with metatarsal dorsiflexion and irritate the interdigital nerve.

History   The patient will typically complain of sharp, burning pain over the plantar aspect of the forefoot. There may be associated paresthesias in the painful area as well as cramping. The patient may describe the sensation of "walking on a marble." The pain is worse in high-heeled street shoes with a narrow toe box and typically relieved with rest and massage of the painful area.

PE   The patient may have localized tenderness over the plantar web space. Motor strength should be normal and sensation may or may not be affected. Squeeze test or Morton's test is performed by firmly squeezing the first and fifth metatarsal heads together with one hand while applying direct pressure to the dorsal and plantar second or third intermetatarsal web space with the other hand. The test is positive when pain is reproduced. Mulder's click is a palpable click that can be felt by the observer during the squeeze test as the metatarsal heads are compressed and the enlarged nerve is displaced inferiorly away from the metatarsal heads.

Imaging/Diagnostic Evaluation   Radiographs are unrevealing. CT has been used; however, it may not be as sensitive as MRI.

Treatment   Initially, appropriately sized, soft-soled shoes with a low heel and wide toe box are recommended for street and dance shoes. A course of physical therapy is generally recommended to include stretching exercises, deep tissue massage, ultrasound, phonophoresis and cryotherapy. Ice and/or NSAIDs may be helpful to reduce inflammation. A plantar pad made of gel or felt can be inserted into the shoe between the affected metatarsals in the affected webspace to aid in spreading the metatarsal heads to relieve compression and irritation of the nerve. If physical therapy and/or padding do not help, consider a corticosteroid–anesthetic injection into the dorsal forefoot proximal to the web space. Care should be taken not to inject the plantar fat pad as necrosis can occur.

If non-operative measures do not adequately relieve the patient's symptoms, consider surgical excision of the common digital nerve. However, risk of surgery includes subsequent development of painful dysesthesias of the toes following excision of the interdigital nerve and possible metatarsal instability depending on the surgical approach.

Case Report A 19-year-old principal female ballet dancer presents to your office complaining of "clicking" in her big toe for the past month and the sensation that her big toe gets "stuck" after which she needs to manually manipulate it. She also complains of pain and swelling posterior to the medial malleolus at the end of jump combinations. She has difficulty rehearsing *pointe* variations involving allegro jumps from flat foot to *pointe*, particularly *échappé* (Figures 1-12).

Diagnosis   Flexor hallucis longus (FHL) tendonitis and trigger toe (hallux saltans)

Epidemiology Occurs most commonly in female classical ballet dancers.

Pathophysiology The FHL acts to plantarflex the hallux and helps plantarflex and stabilize the foot at the subtalar joint. It also helps to prevent pronation of the foot in the *relevé* position. Of the three tendons that run behind the medial malleolus (tibialis posterior (TP), flexor digitorum longus (FDL), FHL), the FHL is the only one that runs through a discrete fibroosseous tunnel. This unique location makes it more susceptible to obstruction along its course through the tunnel.

In dancers, especially in ballet, repetitive transition from the flat foot to the fully plantarflexed *en pointe* position may result in irritation of the FHL

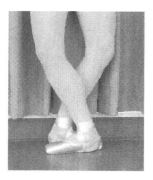

FIGURE 1-12. (**A**) *Échappé* beginning position.

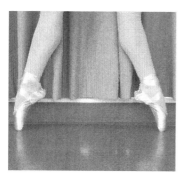

FIGURE 1-12. (**B**) *Échappé en pointe.*

tendon as it passes through the entrance of the FHL tendon sheath, leading to increased likelihood of developing chronic stenosing tenosynovitis. Because the muscle fibers of the FHL tendon are low-lying, they may obstruct smooth movement of the tendon. The FHL tendon may begin to move irregularly through the tunnel, become swollen and nodular and lock distal to the tendon canal near the hallux. This results in the "getting stuck" or "locking" feeling that the dancer describes. In addition to irritation of the tendon, inflammatory changes and swelling may result in pain, typically noticed as the dancer descends from a *demi pointe* to flat foot position. This starts a progressively worsening cycle as the inflamed tendon begins to swell, which causes greater obstruction within the tunnel, which causes more swelling, and more obstruction. Inflammatory changes may ultimately lead to tendon fraying and partial rupture.

History   The patient will typically present complaining of audible "clicking" in the hallux that may or may not be initially painful. This may be accompanied by the toe "getting stuck" or "locking" prior to full dorsiflexion of the FHL. The patient may have to manually release or "unlock" the toe back into normal position. *Grand plié* in fifth position and repetition of *plié* to *relevé* usually exacerbates the pain.

PE   On exam, the patient will typically have tenderness over the **posteromedial** aspect of the ankle (as opposed to **posterolateral** ankle pain, which is more typical of posterior impingement). The patient may have tenderness over three areas that are normally locations of impingement of the FHL tendon—along the course of the tendon through the tunnel posterior to the medial malleolus (**most common**), either under the first metatarsal base where the FHL and FDL tendons cross (knot of Henry) or under the first metatarsal head where the FHL tendon passes between the medial and the lateral sesamoid bones.

When examining the ankle, the knee should be flexed to 90 degrees to relax the gasctrocnemius. **Tomassen's sign** is reflective of FHL tendonitis causing a functional hallux rigidus. This is demonstrated by **decreased** passive dorsiflexion of the first MTP joint with the ankle in **neutral dorsiflexion**, compared to **normal** passive dorsiflexion of the first MTP joint with the ankle in **plantarflexion** (Figures 1-13) [26]. This PROM of hallux dorsiflexion is lost when the ankle is dorsiflexed as the low-lying muscle fibers of the FHL enter the fibro-osseous tunnel and create a temporary functional hallux rigidus. This sign, however, may or may not correlate well with the patient's symptoms.

Pain or triggering with passive ranging of the hallux reflects trigger toe. Resisted hallux plantarflexion may be painful and there may be associated crepitus, triggering, or locking. The nodular thickening can typically be felt as the tendon clicks, snaps, or gets stuck while attempting to pass through the fibro-osseus tunnel.

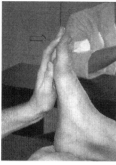

FIGURE 1-13. (**A**) Tomassen's sign.

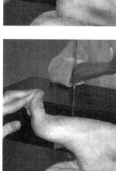

FIGURE 1-13. (**B**) Hallux ROM improved with ankle plantarflexion.

Imaging/Diagnostic Evaluation   AP and lateral radiographs should be obtained to rule out an associated *os trigonum*, which occurs in 8% of the population and reflects a lateral process of the talus that fails to unite. MRI is useful to identify tendon pathology, including tendonitis, tenosynovitis, and tendon tears. Increased fluid in the tendon is often associated with FHL entrapment.

Treatment   Initially, **PRICE** should help decrease the pain and inflammation around the tendon. Physical therapy should focus on soft tissue mobilization, gentle stretching exercises for the FHL prior to and following dance and gastrocnemius strengthening exercises. Also essential is biomechanics education for appropriate rearfoot alignment. If the pain is severe, a course of NSAIDs and immobilization in a removable walker boot may be necessary. Steroid injections have been traditionally contraindicated secondary to proximity of the neurovascular bundle; however, recent advances using musculoskeletal ultrasound to visualize the area have allowed skilled sonographers to inject corticosteroid into the FHL sheath as a therapeutic option.

If a course of conservative management with PRICE and physical therapy do not relieve the patient's symptoms, surgery may be considered to incise the stenosing entrance of the FHL sheath and repair or debride the FHL tendon. Tenosynovectomy is often required. Arthroscopic release of the FHL is currently not recommended [27].

Case Report   A 30-year-old female modern dancer presents to your office complaining of pain over the plantar aspect of her heel, especially when walking barefoot and when she takes her first step getting out of bed in the morning. She denies associated trauma or recent increase in dance activity.

Diagnosis   Plantar fasciitis

Epidemiology   Common injury of the hindfoot.

Pathophysiology   The plantar fascia is located superficial to the intrinsic foot muscles and deep to the plantar fat pad, providing the dense connective tissue over the sole of the foot. It attaches to the anterior calcaneus proximally and to the plantar aspect of the phalanges distally and is involved in distributing the forces to the plantar foot during heel strike and normal ambulation. In dancers, repetitive jumping, inadequate shock absorption on a poorly reinforced floor, and prolonged standing can lead to irritation of the plantar aponeurosis with subsequent microtrauma and degenerative changes in the fascia.

A concept known as the **windlass effect** was first described by Cailliet in 1980, describing the mechanism by which the plantar fascia provides static support for the longitudinal arch of the foot during weight bearing and helps provide shock absorption during foot strike [28]. During gait in the heel-off phase, the plantar fascia is taut and under tension, providing a source of potential energy. During the toe-off phase, the plantar fascia effectively shortens with hallux dorsiflexion and provides propulsive motion as kinetic energy. The repetitive high energy forces created during pronation and supination during the gait cycle increase tension on the plantar fascia. When a poorly aligned foot or one with weak supporting muscles is subject to these high energy forces repeatedly, increased tissue stress occurs with greater likelihood of injury [29].

History   Dancers will often describe pain after a full day of rehearsals and/ or classes in which they have been jumping and/or spending a great deal of time on their feet. Symptoms can be worse after dancing on a hardwood floor that is not sprung, or any other hard surface not adequately reinforced for shock absorption. They will typically report plantar heel pain when walking or dancing following rest and/or **in the morning when taking a first step out of bed**.

PE   Physical examination of the foot should include palpation of the medial heel and length of the plantar fascia, including the arch of the foot. The patient may have an isolated point of maximal tenderness in this area or may have more diffuse pain along the proximal attachment of the plantar fascia to the anterior calcaneus. However, tenderness to palpation should be specific to the plantar fascia. Tenderness at the plantar heel pad is more indicative of heel pad inflammation and requires different treatment. Forceful dorsiflexion of the toes or standing in the *demi pointe* position often exacerbates the pain, as these maneuvers tighten the plantar fascia. Conversely, returning the toes to neutral position or into plantarflexion, as in full *pointe*, should decrease the pain.

Imaging/Diagnostic Evaluation   Radiographs may be obtained to rule out other etiologies when initial management has failed. MRI is also typically reserved for confirmation of diagnosis in refractory cases.

Treatment   Initially, **PRICE** should form the mainstay of therapy. If pain persists, a course of NSAIDs may be helpful. Physical therapy should focus on releasing tight tissue, heel cord stretching, strengthening and fascial stretching. An **overnight splint** can provide gentle stretching to the plantar aspect of the foot for a longer duration, but may not be well tolerated by patients. A carbon footplate beneath the insole of a street or dance shoe or a rocker bottom soled shoe can help minimize MTP joint dorsiflexion and inadequate MTP joint dorsiflexion during push-off.

Corticosteroid injections into the plantar fascia should typically be avoided. Injection into the plantar fat pad can result in atrophy of the area and loss of significant normal shock absorption from the forces of regular walking and dance activity. A rare but serious risk includes plantar fascia rupture. Also, oral steroids are typically not recommended as local absorption of the steroid by the plantar fascia is low secondary to poor vascularization of the plantar fascia. Extracorporeal shock wave therapy has also been used in patients with associated heel spurs although with mixed results [30].

Surgical options should be considered only as a last resort. Operative treatment would typically involve division of the central portion of the plantar aponeurosis, partial fasciectomy, and/or neurolysis of the abductor digiti quinti nerve. Surgery is only very rarely indicated, with risks including development of a painful neuroma with severe residual pain that may be worse than the preoperative pain.

Case Report   A 25-year-old modern dancer presents to your office complaining of left foot pain that has persisted over the past 8–9 months. She has history of two prior sprains on the same ankle, one mild and one severe. Her current pain has persisted longer than her first sprains.

Diagnosis   **Sinus tarsi syndrome or sinus tarsitis**

Epidemiology   An uncommon diagnosis to suspect when a sprained ankle does not heal.

Pathophysiology   The sinus tarsi originates as a laterally located groove bordered superiorly by the talus and inferiorly by the calcaneus and travels medially to form the canalis tarsi. A number of ligaments traverse its borders and may be involved in an ankle sprain. Biomechanically, when the patient pronates the foot, the soft tissue within the sinus tarsi is compressed, increasing the pressure within it as well as the pressure in the subtalar joint. When severe, hyperpronation can obliterate the sinus tarsi. Over time, soft tissue within the sinus tarsi that may have been initially inflamed following trauma, associated with a partially torn ligament or chronically compressed in individuals with overpronated feet, may develop scar tissue and associated chronic inflammation.

History   When a dancer presents with history of trauma and an ankle sprain that is not healing, suspect this diagnosis as the cause. The patient will typically complain of deep lateral hindfoot pain, worse with passive ankle inversion or eversion. The patient may feel that the ankle is loose or unstable, with pain worse while standing and walking on uneven surfaces.

PE   Careful examination of the foot will likely reveal tenderness over the lateral hindfoot region overlying the tarsal sinus. There may be associated ligamentous instability.

Imaging/Diagnostic Evaluation   Standard AP and lateral radiographs of the foot will rule out any underlying bony pathology including arthritis, fracture, or dislocation. Injection of local anesthetic into the sinus tarsi with subsequent relief of the patient's pain is a commonly used diagnostic technique. MRI can also better visualize the presence of soft tissue inflammation within the sinus or deep to it, within the canalis tarsi.

Treatment   **PRICE** forms the initial mainstay of treatment. Bracing and custom molded ankle orthotics that limit subtalar joint range of motion are helpful. If the pain persists, a local corticosteroid injection can be used to help reduce inflammation and pain. Procedures to ablate the nociceptive nerve endings found in the canalis tarsi include chemical and thermal ablation. Chemical ablation has been utilized with serial injections of alcohol, whereas thermal ablation freezes the involved nociceptive nerve endings. Arthroscopic evaluation and debridement of the sinus tarsi is also an option if the above treatment measures fail [31].

References

1. Gould N, Schneider W, Ashikaga T. Epidemiological survey of foot problems in the continental US 1978–79. Foot Ankle 1980; 1(1): 8–10.
2. Shereff MJ, Baumhauer JF. Hallux rigidus and osteoarthrosis of the first metatarsophalangeal joint. J Bone Joint Surg Am 1998; 80(6): 898–908.
3. Mulier T, Steenwerckx A, Thienpont E. Results after cheilectomy in athletes with hallux rigidus. Foot Ankle Int 1999; 20(4): 232.
4. Fetzer GB, Wright RW. Metatarsal shaft fractures and fractures of the proximal fifth metatarsal. Clin Sports Med 2006; 25: 139–50.
5. O'Malley MJ, Hamilton WG, Munyak JM. Fractures of the distal shaft of the fifth metatarsal: "Dancer's Fracture." Am J Sports Med 1996; 24(2): 240–47.
6. Dameron TB. Fractures and anatomic variations of the proximal portion of the fifth metatarsal. J Bone Joint Surg Am 1972; 57(6): 788–92.
7. Macintyre J, Joy E. Foot and ankle injuries in dance. Clin Sports Med 2000 19(2): 351–68.
8. Rosenberg GA, Sferra JJ. Treatment strategies for acute fractures and nonunions of the proximal fifth metatarsal. J Am Acad Orthop Surg 2000; 8(5): 332–38.
9. Wright RW, Fischer DA, Shively RA et al. Refracture of proximal fifth metatarsal (Jones) fracture after intramedullary screw fixation in athletes. Am J Sports Med 2000; 28: 732–36.
10. Brown SR, Bennett CH. Management of proximal fifth metatarsal fractures in the athlete. Curr Opin Ortho 2005; 16(2): 95–99.
11. Myburgh KH, Hutchins J, Fataar AB et al. Low bone mineral density is an etiologic factor for stress fractures in athletes. Ann Int Med 1990; 113: 754–59.
12. Weinfeld S, Haddad S, Myerson M. Metatarsal stress fractures. Clin Sports Med 1997; 16(2): 319–38.
13. Torg JS, Balduini FC, Zelko RR et al. Fractures of the base of the fifth metatarsal distal to the tuberosity. J Bone Joint Surg Am 1984; 66(2): 209–14.
14. Micheli LJ, Sohn RS, Solomon R. Stress fractures of the second metatarsal involving Lisfranc's joint in ballet dancers. A new overuse injury of the foot. J Bone Joint Surg 1985; 67(9): 1372–75.
15. Harrington T, Crichton KJ, Anderson IF. Overuse ballet injury to the base of the second metatarsal – a diagnostic problem. Am J Sports Med 1993; 21: 591–98.
16. Mullen JE, O'Malley MJ. Sprains – residual instability of subtalar, Lisfranc joints and turf toe. Clin Sports Med 2004; 23(1): 97–121.
17. Ameres MJ. Navicular fracture. Emedicine: http://www.emedicine.com/sports/topic85.htm
18. Drez D, Young JC, Waldman D et al. Nonoperative treatment of double lateral ligament tears of the ankle. Am J Sports Med 1982; 10: 197–200.
19. Rosenfield JS, Trepman E. Treatment of sesamoid disorders with a rocker sole shoe modification. Foot Ankle Int 2000; 21(11): 914–15.
20. McBryde AM, Anderson RB. Sesamoid foot problems in the athlete. Clin Sports Med 1988; 7(1): 51–60.
21. Childs, SG. The pathogenesis and biomechanics of turf toe. Ortho Nurs 2006; 25(4): 276–80.
22. Title CI, Katchis SD. Traumatic foot and ankle injuries in the athlete. Ortho Clin N Am 2002; 33: 587–98.
23. Ohlson B. Turf toe. Emedicine: http://www.emedicine.com/orthoped/topic572.htm
24. Kadel N. Foot and ankle injuries in dance. Phys Med Reh Clin N Am 2006; 17(4): 813–26.
25. Marshall P, Hamilton WG. Cuboid subluxation in ballet dancers. Am J Sports Med 1992; 20: 169–75.

26. Tomassen E. Disease and injuries of ballet dancers 1982; Arhus, Denmark. Universitetsforlaget I Arhus.
27. Hamilton WG, Geppert MJ, Thompson FM. Pain in the posterior aspect of the ankle in dancers. Differential diagnosis and operative treatment. J Bone Joint Surg 1996; 78-A(10): 1491–1500.
28. Cailliet R. Foot and ankle pain. Philadelphia, PA. FA Davis Publications, 2nd edition, Nov 1982.
29. Bolgla LA, Malone TR. Plantar fasciitis and the windlass mechanism: A biomechanical link to clinical practice. J Athl Train 2004; 39(1): 77–82.
30. Pommering TL, Kluchurosky L, Hall SL. Ankle and foot injuries in pediatric and adult athletes. Prim Care: Clin Off Prac 2005; 32(1): 133–61.
31. Kuwada GT. Long-term retrospective analysis of the treatment of sinus tarsi syndrome. J Foot Ankle Surg 1994; 33(1): 28–9.

2
Ankle Injuries

Case Report   A 22-year-old *corps de ballet* dancer is rehearsing an adagio movement and complains that she cannot fully *plié* on her right side. Range of motion beyond the *demi plié* position is painful on the right.

Diagnosis   Anterior impingement syndrome

Epidemiology   Commonly occurs in ballet dancers, more often following severe or multiple ankle sprains.

Pathophysiology   Ballet dancers commonly perform repetitive ankle dorsiflexion in the positions of *demi* and *grand plié* (Figures 2-1). *Demi plié* is not only a component of the basic dance vocabulary but also forms the beginning and ending positions of jumps or transitions from one movement to another. Repetitive ankle dorsiflexion may lead to anterior impingement between the tibia (anterior lip) and talus (neck), resulting in bony formation (osteophytes) along the anterior aspect of the ankle. The bony reactive formation can compress the soft tissue of the anterior ankle, impinge the capsule, and subsequently cause pain. Irritation in this area is associated with an inflammatory reaction and swelling of the anterior ankle joint. Repetitive excessive ankle dorsiflexion causing pain can be associated with an anterior bony spur as well as an atypically shaped talar dome.

History   The patient usually recounts anterolateral ankle pain reproduced by *demi plié*. He or she may complain that their ankle gets "stuck," feels awkward, or unsteady in the *plié* position.

PE   Clicking or crepitus is common. The patient may have pain on palpation along the anterolateral joint line, although anteromedial joint line tenderness may also be felt. There may be associated swelling and/or limited active range of motion of the ankle. Pain will typically be elicited with active dorsiflexion of the ankle and may be associated with pain with passive ankle

From: *Musculoskeletal Medicine: Essential Dance Medicine*
By A. Bracilović, DOI 10.1007/978-1-59745-546-6_2,
© Humana Press, a part of Springer Science+Business Media, LLC 2009

(A)

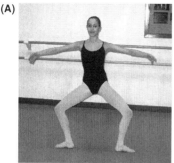

FIGURE 2-1. (**A**) *Demi plié* in second position.

(B)

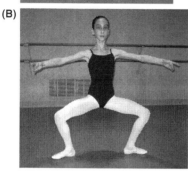

FIGURE 2-1. (**B**) *Grand plié* in second position.

dorsiflexion. Osteophytic changes may be palpated while holding the ankle in slight plantarflexion.

Imaging/Diagnostic Evaluation Although anterior impingement can occur without bone spurs and/or osteophyte formation, imaging is recommended to rule out other causes of anterior ankle pain and reveal any associated joint pathology. Standard weight bearing ankle radiographs can demonstrate arthritis, fracture, osteochondritis dissecans lesion, mortise disruption, and/or tibiotalar joint space narrowing. Lateral views can reveal talar and tibial osteophytes associated with anterior impingement. On MRI, T1 and proton density axial views can demonstrate soft tissue impingement, including thickened synovium in the anterior lateral joint space or hypertrophy of the anterior talofibular ligament [1].

Treatment PRICE and treatment with NSAIDs can help alleviate acute pain and reduce swelling around the ankle joint. Initially, deep *pliés* should be avoided. The dancer can also try using quarter to half-inch heel lifts to decrease the amount of ankle dorsiflexion in class and normal walking throughout the day. If non-operative intervention does not relieve the pain, arthroscopic surgery may be considered to remove either the impinging soft tissue and/or bony growth, including scar tissue and tibial and/or talar osteophytes [2].

Case Report   A 22-year-old principal ballet dancer presents to your office complaining of pain and clicking when she points her foot and attempts *relevé en pointe*. The pain is over the posterolateral aspect of her ankle and is worst while in full *pointe*.

Diagnosis   Posterior impingement syndrome, also known as "dancer's heel"

Epidemiology   Common in female ballet dancers dancing *en pointe*.

Pathophysiology   An accessory bone called an *os trigonum* may be found just posterior to the talus in 2.5–14% of normal feet. Usually, this accessory bone causes little to no symptoms in non-dancers. In ballet dancers, however, who often utilize the fully plantarflexed position when on full *pointe*, an *os trigonum* can cause significant pain and discomfort by compressing the soft tissue in the posterior ankle. The *os trigonum* can vary in size and arises from a separate ossification center posterior to the lateral tubercle or the posterior talar process. It may fuse with the lateral tubercle or remain as a separate small bone. Inflammation in and around the ossicle as well as the FHL tendon can result. Also, if the ballet dancer has significant ligamentous laxity and/or the pointed foot is too far forward in the pointe shoe, the talar dome and surrounding soft tissue can be compressed between the tibia and the calcaneus, causing posterior impingement. Overuse of positions placing the transverse tarsal (Chopart's) joint into plantarflexion in tap (double toe stance) (Figures 2-2) can also predispose to posterior impingement.

History   Often, the patient will report pain in the posterolateral aspect of the ankle with episodes of repeated plantarflexion onto *pointe* and frequent *relevé*. The patient will typically complain of **posterolateral** ankle pain that is worse with ankle plantarflexion. The pain may be associated with swelling and/or tenderness in the posterior aspect of the ankle. The pain is worse with forced passive plantarflexion of the ankle, known as the "plantarflexion sign," which has been characterized as the hallmark of posterior impingement [3].

PE   The **plantarflexion sign** involves the examiner holding the heel of the symptomatic foot in one hand and forcefully plantarflexing the forefoot (Figure 2-3). The sign is considered **positive** when this motion is painful and is indicative of posterior impingement. The sign is helpful to rule out other conditions and should be **negative** with Achilles, FHL, and peroneal tendonitis.

Imaging/Diagnostic Evaluation   On plain radiographs, an *os trigonum* appears as dense cortical bone with smooth edges. It is important to rule out a fracture of the lateral tubercle when a separate bone is seen. A **lateral radiograph with the foot in 15 degrees of internal rotation** moves the fibula anteriorly to better visualize an *os trigonum*, if present. This is a helpful additional radiographic image. MRI is useful in identifying soft tissue and

(A)

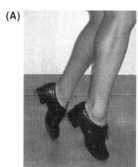

(B)

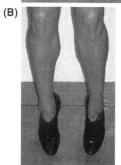

(C)

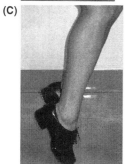

FIGURE 2-2. (**A–C**) Double toe stance in tap.

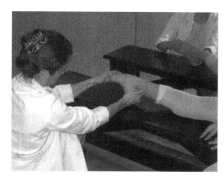

FIGURE 2-3. Plantarflexion sign.

bony pathology, including fracture of the *os trigonum*, FHL tenosynovitis, talocalcaneal synovitis, or bone marrow edema. A trial intra-articular injection of lidocaine can help distinguish between ankle and subtalar pain.

Treatment   Initially, **PRICE** should help reduce the pain and inflammation. Anti-inflammatory medications including NSAIDs may be helpful to reduce the soft tissue swelling. Physical therapy should focus on stretching the posterior soft tissue of the Achilles tendon and gastrocnemius and soleus muscles. A trial intra-articular anesthetic injection into the posterior aspect of the tibial talar joint may be helpful. If injection of intra-articular lidocaine alleviates the pain, consider corticosteroid injection into the affected area.

If the pain does not respond to initial conservative management, surgery may need to be considered to remove the *os trigonum* and impinging soft tissues. Although both posterolateral and posteromedial approaches have been recommended, the posteromedial approach is a safer approach to avoid both the neurovascular bundle as well as damage to the adjacent FHL, especially if release of an associated FHL tendonitis/tenosynovitis is required. Although arthroscopic excision of the *os trigonum* has been reported, it is not recommended at this time for the dancer.

Case Report   A 16-year-old "Riverdance" performer comes to your office complaining of pain in her lower calf and heel, especially in the morning and after a day of dancing. She has stiffness in the morning and often has swelling in the same area at the end of the day, worse after jump combinations.

Diagnosis   Achilles tendonitis and tendinosis

Epidemiology   Higher frequency in jumpers and runners, following acute changes in rehearsal and/or activity schedule.

Pathophysiology   The Achilles tendon is the body's longest tendon and connects the calf muscles to the calcaneus. It allows plantarflexion of the foot and helps the foot *relevé* into *demi pointe* and full *pointe* positions. It can sustain forces greater than 1000 pounds, and as a result of its frequent use and overuse is often susceptible to inflammation in dancers, gymnasts, runners, and cyclists. Intense training over a short period of time, lack of natural flexibility of the calf muscles and returning to dance after an extended absence all increase the risk of injury. Dancing, especially jumping, on hardwood or non-sprung floors in shoes with insufficient shock absorbance is also a risk factor. During allegro jumps, the gastrocnemius is eccentrically most active when it absorbs impact from the ground on initial contact. This prevents forward motion of the leg on landing from jumps.

The development of Achilles tendon pain can be attributed to processes that have been distinguished as two entities: tendonitis and tendinosis. Tendonitis describes a predominant process of inflammation, whereas tendinosis is associated with degenerative changes that can occur without histologic signs of inflammation. Tendonitis involves peritendinous inflammation that does not typically progress to degenerative tendinosis. When evaluated histologically, collagen and related fiber cells comprising the Achilles tendon that reflect degeneration, disorganization, and scarring are associated with tendinosis.

History   The patient may present after overusing the calf muscles for a prolonged period of time in rehearsals or during summer intensives. The pain is typically located in the posterior heel and/or lower calf and is worse during jumps.

PE   There is often tenderness to palpation of the tendon from 1 to 5 cm proximal to the calcaneus. It may be possible to palpate a nodule or fusiform swelling in this area. As opposed to an Achilles tendon rupture, no defect should be felt and Thompson's test will be **negative** (Figure 2-4). Active resisted plantarflexion may be painful, as well as passive ankle dorsiflexion. By gently palpating or squeezing the Achilles tendon while the patient actively plantarflexes and dorsiflexes the ankle, crepitus can be felt.

Imaging/Diagnostic Evaluation   Imaging is often not needed for the diagnosis of Achilles tendonitis, but may be helpful in narrowing the differential

FIGURE 2-4. Negative Thompson's test.

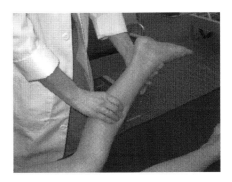

diagnosis and should be ordered accordingly. Plain radiographs of the ankle joint may show calcification of the distal Achilles in tendonitis. MRI is useful in distinguishing tendonitis from tears within the tendon itself.

Treatment   The goal of immediate treatment is to reduce pain and inflammation and involves **PRICE** and physical therapy. The level of patient's pain should direct the intensity of allowable exercises, with the goal of pain free activity at all times. Dancers, especially, need to be aware of their limits and allow only pain-free range of motion when stretching the Achilles with active ankle dorsiflexion and calf stretching.

The intermediate phase of therapy should introduce strengthening exercises, specifically eccentric exercises for the gastrocnemius and soleus, slowly and gradually. Cryotherapy, ultrasound, electrical stimulation, and neuromuscular control programs are introduced as tolerated to reduce pain, inflammation, and edema. An orthotic such as a heel lift can be placed in the street shoe to relieve tension on the tendon or if structural imbalances are present.

For chronic or recurrent pain, an overnight splint may help improve ankle dorsiflexion range of motion. If the tendonitis is resistant to treatment, casting may be used as a last resort, in the form of an air cast walking brace combined with a heel lift. Although the brace immobilizes the ankle and reduces stretching of the Achilles tendon prior to push-off, the brace should be removed 4–6 times per day to prevent stiffness from developing in the joint.

In the maintenance phase, increasing amounts of stress are provided to encourage collagen to form and healing to continue. Stretching and active resistive range of motion exercises are progressively increased in intensity and may include selected Pilates exercises and/or pool therapy. Dancers should be trained in a structured home exercise program to maintain strength and range of motion, as well as to reduce the risk of repeat injury.

Medical therapy for Achilles tendonitis involves the use of anti-inflammatory medications, most often in the form of NSAIDs. Always keep in mind possible side effects, including liver damage from acetaminophen, gastrointestinal bleeding, and renal damage from COX-2 inhibitors. Steroid injections should typically be avoided in Achilles tendonitis secondary to risk of tendon weakening and potential rupture [4].

Surgery is rarely required for debridement of recalcitrant Achilles tendinosis and should be considered only after greater than 6 months of failed conservative management.

Case Report   A 36-year-old female ballet dancer presents to your office after experiencing acute pain in her posterior right ankle during a jump combination in ballet class. She was attempting a *changement de pieds* (Figure 2-5) from fifth position when she felt and heard a "popping" feeling in the back of her heel, as if someone hit her in the ankle. She had immediate difficulty with *relevé* and walking.

Diagnosis   **Achilles tendon rupture**

Epidemiology   Occurs more often in older dancers, 30–50 years old.

Pathophysiology   It has been shown that most Achilles tendon ruptures occur within a relatively avascular zone, approximately 2–6 cm proximal to the calcaneal insertion [5]. Some patients may have history of prior injury to the Achilles tendon and the tendon may rupture acutely in the setting of chronically weakened fibrotic tissue.

History   The patient will often report an abrupt repetitive motion such as take-off from a jump as in an Allegro combination, where an eccentric load was rapidly applied to a tendon in tension with a dorsiflexed ankle and extended knee. The patient will often report feeling and/or hearing a "pop" or feeling that they were struck in the posterior ankle from behind. The patient will often experience acute pain that may subside, but loss of function will persist.

PE   There is often acute pain and the patient cannot adequately plantarflex the ankle or rise in *relevé*. Ecchymosis and swelling are often diffuse. On palpation, the patient will have a tendon gap and a positive Thompson sign with lack of passive ankle plantarflexion when the calf is manually squeezed. The patient will be unable to *relevé* on the affected leg and may or may not have decreased resisted active plantarflexion strength. It is important to have the patient actively *relevé* as strong, muscular dancers may be able to maintain adequate plantarflexion strength assuming their unaffected flexor tendons are intact, including the FDL, FHL, peroneus longus and brevis, plantaris, and tibialis posterior.

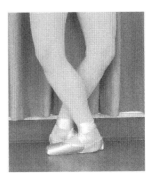

FIGURE 2-5. *Changement de pieds.*

Imaging/Diagnostic Evaluation   Although the diagnosis is most often clinical, MRI is recommended when considering operative intervention.

Treatment   In dancers who wish to resume activity as soon as possible, early surgical intervention is most often recommended. It has been shown that early operative management is associated with a decreased incidence of repeat rupture [6].

Physical therapy emphasizing **early mobilization** has been associated with better tendon healing, reduced rate of adhesions, and improved tendon strength [7]. Following surgical repair, initial immobilization for 7–10 days in a plantarflexed position in a short leg walking boot is recommended. Active dorsiflexion exercises should be encouraged with a dorsiflexion stop. Progressive decrease of plantarflexed immobilization should occur, with removal of increasing wedges. Weight bearing is usually restricted for 2–8 weeks. The walking boot is removed at 6 weeks and the patient can walk with a heel pad for the following 3 months. Range of motion exercises are emphasized for the first 2–3 months, followed by strengthening exercises for the next 3 months. Usually following 6 months, the patient is allowed to return to dance.

Case Report   A 24-year-old ballet dancer is in training for the annual performance of the Nutcracker. She is practicing an allegro combination at the end of a long day of rehearsal. In the middle of a jump combination, she missteps the landing and falls onto her foot in an inverted, supinated position. She experiences immediate pain over the lateral aspect of her foot and hears a "popping" sound.

Diagnosis   Lateral ankle sprain

Epidemiology   Most common ankle injury in dancers.

Pathophysiology   The dancer is able to normally maintain ankle stability in various plantarflexed positions in *demi pointe* and full *pointe* as a result of the static and dynamic stabilizers of the ankle. In the full *pointe* position, the ankle is relatively stable at the subtalar joint as the calcaneus locks against the posterior aspect of the tibia. When the dancer descends from full *pointe* into *demi pointe* or with loss of balance, this joint stability is lost and greater pressure is placed on the dynamic stabilizers of the ankle, mainly provided by three ligaments, to stabilize the joint. The anterior talofibular ligament (ATFL), calcaneofibular ligament (CFL), and posterior talofibular ligament (PTFL) stabilize the ankle as well as help maintain proprioception. The ATFL and the peroneal muscles predominantly stabilize the ankle in this position. Of the three stabilizing ligaments, the ATFL is actually the weakest and most frequently injured. The CFL provides subtalar stability and is most taut in dorsiflexion, whereas the PTFL is most taut in severe dorsiflexion. The PTFL is most rarely injured as it is the strongest ligament.

With increased dorsiflexion, the ankle becomes more susceptible to inversion injury. The anatomy of the talus bone is such that it is wider anteriorly and narrower posteriorly, resulting in an inherent instability when the ankle is in a plantarflexed position. Weak and tired peroneal muscles also predispose the dancer to an ankle sprain in this position.

A grade I ankle sprain typically reflects a stretched or partially torn ATFL and intact CFL with no associated mechanical instability or significant increase in laxity. A grade II sprain reflects a complete ATFL tear and partial tear of the CFL, with increased medial tenderness and mild to moderate instability. A grade III tear reflects a complete tear of the ATFL, CFL and partial tear of the PTFL, with significant tenderness, swelling, and difficulty bearing weight both medially and laterally.

History   There are multiple risk factors in dancers for this very common injury. Previous ankle sprains, fatigue, returning to stage too quickly before an injury has had enough time to heal, inadequate rehabilitation and poor landing technique are frequently associated risk factors. Specific steps such as entrechat six and other components of allegro combinations in ballet as well as certain positions in tap (wings) (Figures 2-6) that are associated with difficult landings are also commonly cited preceding ankle sprains in dancers [8].

(A)

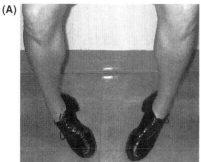

FIGURE 2-6. (**A**) Wing mid stance.

(B)

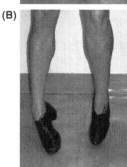

FIGURE 2-6. (**B**) Toe stance wing.

The patient will typically report injury following landing from a jump with the ankle in plantarflexion, incorrectly either onto the ground with loss of balance or onto an object, other dancer, piece of equipment, etc. Ambulation and weight bearing are progressively more difficult for grades I and II and the patient is typically not able to weight bear with grade III sprains.

PE Full examination of the foot and ankle may be limited secondary to pain and swelling, if the patient presents a few hours after the injury. Typically, there is lateral tenderness over the fibular insertion of the ATFL and if the injury is more severe, over the calcaneal insertion of the CFL if it is involved as well. The patient will usually have a positive anterior drawer test, which assesses the integrity of the ATFL. The examiner should stabilize the distal leg in one hand and anteriorly translate the heel with the foot in a relaxed plantarflexed position (about 20 degrees) (Figure 2-7). The test is positive if there is a greater than 3–5 mm difference in laxity between the affected and unaffected side with no clear endpoint on the affected side. The talar tilt test, also known as the varus stress test or inversion stress test, assesses the integrity of the ATFL and CFL. It is positive with increased excursion of the inverted heel while the ankle is dorsiflexed as compared to the opposite side (Figure 2-8). Specifically, greater than 23 degrees of angulation or more than 10 degrees of difference when compared to the

FIGURE 2-7. Ankle anterior drawer test.

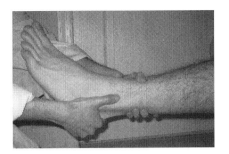

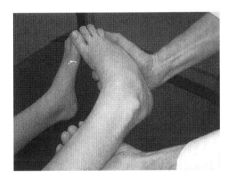

FIGURE 2-8. Talar tilt test.

unaffected side has been associated with complete ATFL and CFL tears [9]. Mild to moderate joint instability is typically associated with a positive anterior drawer test and negative talar tilt test, whereas severe joint instability is associated with positive anterior drawer and talar tilt tests.

Imaging/Diagnostic Evaluation   Any patient with difficulty bearing weight or experiencing pain over the base of the fifth metatarsal, medial and lateral malleoli, navicular bone or posterior inferior 4 inches of the tibia and fibular should have anterior-posterior (AP), lateral and mortise radiographs of the ankle initially to rule out fractures, osteochondral, and/or joint abnormalities. Also, an AP radiograph of the foot should be obtained to rule out anterior calcaneal injury or a fifth metatarsal fracture.

Treatment   Initially, **PRICE** should be instituted as soon as possible following injury. Depending on the grade of injury, the degree of immobilization needed for the ankle will vary. **Grade I and II** sprains typically need a gel-cast or air-cast ankle brace. **Grade III** sprains may require short leg brace for no longer than 2 weeks, followed by an air cast. Crutches or a cane are utilized for weight bearing as tolerated.

Pursuing and completing a full course of physical therapy is important with ankle sprains given the likelihood of recurrence once the initial sprain occurs. Therapy should focus on improving strength and balance for return to dance activities. Dancers with grade I or II sprains should be able to return to dance within 1–2 weeks. Patients are typically allowed to return to dance if they can single leg hop for 10 consecutive jumps and fully squat [D. J. Rose, personal communication]. A well-structured functional rehabilitation program is essential to restore the dancer's full range of motion, endurance, strength, balance, and proprioception.

After a grade III injury, PRICE is especially important and protection of the ankle should continue for up to 6 months following return to dance activity. For dancers, surgery is a last resort option as dynamic function is sacrificed for mechanical stability. Surgery typically results in increased recovery time, time away from classes and off stage, muscle disuse, atrophy, and subsequent loss of range of motion. This is often an unacceptable outcome for professional dancers. Only if the dancer has chronic complaints of ankle instability that interfere with ability to dance despite conservative management should surgery be considered. The modified Brostrøm procedure has been performed with success [10], but surgery for dancers is always a last resort option.

Case Report   An 11-year-old boy active in Irish dancing and gymnastics presents to your office complaining of right heel pain when running and jumping during classes and practice sessions. The pain started gradually and is better with rest but has continued to bother him over the past 2–3 months.

Diagnosis   Calcaneal apophysitis (Sever's disease)

Epidemiology   More common in active 10–12-year-old boys.

Pathophysiology   First described in 1912 by Dr. J.W. Sever as inflammation of the calcaneal apophysis, Sever's disease is a type of osteochondrosis seen in children and adolescents. The calcaneal apophysis appears in 9–10-year-old boys, 7–9-year-old girls and normally ossifies by 17–18 years old. During puberty, microfractures may develop around the growth line as a result of repetitive shear stress over this susceptible, growing area that is weakened from the tension of the Achilles tendon, gastrocnemius, and soleus and the newly forming calcified cartilage.

History   The patient will typically present complaining of posterior heel pain, difficulty walking, and may have associated swelling in the painful area. The pain is worse with running, jumping, and improves with rest. The pain is usually gradual and does not bother the patient at night.

PE   The patient will typically have posterior heel tenderness over the insertion of the Achilles. Active and forced ankle dorsiflexion may be painful.

Imaging/Diagnostic Evaluation   Standard radiographs are useful to rule out fracture or bony lesions. They can demonstrate fragments and sclerosis of the apophysis, however, do not provide pathognomonic findings of apophysitis.

Treatment   Initial treatment includes **PRICE** and reducing the amount of running and jumping in dance or gymnastic activities. A specific functional rehabilitation program should focus on stretching of the Achilles tendon, gastrocnemius, and soleus complex and strengthening of the associated muscles. A half-inch heel lift can help reduce tension on the Achilles tendon-apophysial attachment. NSAIDs may be necessary for pain relief. Local corticosteroid injections to this area are contraindicated secondary to the risk of Achilles tendon rupture. For severe pain, casting in mild equinus may be necessary for a 2–3 week period [11].

Case Report   A 35-year-old female former professional figure skater presents to your office complaining of pain over the medial arch of her foot, worse after practice sessions and associated with swelling behind her right medial malleolus.

Diagnosis   Posterior tibial tendonitis

Epidemiology   Often misdiagnosed and underreported dance injury.

Pathophysiology   The posterior tibialis muscle originates from the interosseous membrane and the posterior surfaces of the tibia and fibula and inserts on the tuberosity of the navicular, cuneiform, and cuboid bones as well as the bases of the second, third, and fourth metatarsals. Its functions are to plantarflex the ankle and invert the foot. If dancers force turn-out from their feet, excess pronation will occur, placing increased strain on the posterior tibialis muscle. Furthermore, ballet aesthetics emphasizes the appearance of a "winged" foot that plantarflexes, abducts, and everts the foot, excessively stretching the posterior tibialis tendon (Figure 2-9). In addition to the strain of ballet, any premorbid structural causes of biomechanical misalignment, such as unilateral or bilateral pes planus or an accessory navicular bone may further increase the risk of poor rearfoot alignment and subsequent posterior tibialis tendon strain. Tenosynovitis more often than a posterior tibialis tendon tear is the underlying pathology in dancers.

History   The patient will often report a history of increased time spent in training, either in classes or in rehearsals. Often, the activity will involve increased frequency of jump combinations. External factors such as a new dance floor lacking adequate shock absorption may also be a contributing factor.

PE   The patient will typically have tenderness to palpation over the posterior tibialis tendon posterior and inferior to the medial malleolus. There may be associated swelling in the same area. With significant symptoms, the patient will typically not be able to *relevé* onto the affected foot or may do so with resultant pain in the medial ankle. Resisted ankle plantarflexion and

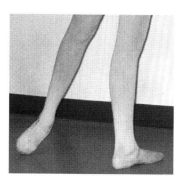

FIGURE 2-9. Winging of the right foot.

inversion are also usually painful and/or weak. For those patients who overpronate, they will also typically demonstrate the "too many toes" sign, initially described by Johnson [12].

A test that can reflect early posterior tibialis tendon dysfunction has been described as the first metatarsal rise sign, where the head of the first metatarsal rises with passive heel varus [13].

Imaging/Diagnostic Evaluation   Standard AP and lateral weight bearing radiographs of the symptomatic and asymptomatic foot should be obtained, but may initially be normal. As symptoms progress, the talonavicular joint may sublux as the navicular bone rotates laterally on the talus and the longitudinal arch may collapse. MRI is useful to evaluate any bony, tendinous, or soft tissue pathology.

Treatment   Patients with acute tenosynovitis can initially be immobilized in a short walking boot. Custom molded orthotics can provide corrective support for patients who overpronate. A functional rehabilitation program that focuses on stretching of the Achilles tendon and gastrocnemius-soleus complex as well as strengthening of the posterior tibialis muscle are important to return the patient to dance activity.

Surgical exploration and debridement of the posterior tibialis tendon is an available option typically reserved for non-operative treatment failures. It involves excision of any inflamed tenosynovium with debridement and repair of any partial tendon tears. Post-operatively, patients are allowed to ambulate in a short walking boot or cast for 4–6 weeks, combined with a functional rehabilitation program that progresses to return to full activity approximately 8–12 weeks following surgery [14].

Case Report A 13-year-old female figure skater presents to your office complaining of pain and swelling behind her right lateral malleolus that is worse after skating practice. She occasionally feels a sharp "pinch" over the same area.

Diagnosis Peroneal tendonitis

Epidemiology Common in young dancers who have not yet developed sufficient strength for *pointe.*

Pathophysiology In ballet, the desired externally rotated positions of the legs often concentrically contract the peroneal muscles. Over time, chronic shortening of these muscles can irritate and inflame the peroneus long and brevis tendons in their sheaths. Peroneal tendonitis arises most commonly as an overuse injury following repetitive jump combinations that require abrupt changes in direction or frequent "push off" as seen in ice skating. Chronically, the peroneal tendons can be damaged with recurrent lateral ankle sprains that ultimately lead to small tendon tears. Inflammatory proteins and fluid surround the tendons, increasing pressure in the space between the tendon and the sheath, resulting in pain, swelling, and ultimately weakness.

History Dancers who are performing jump or allegro combinations in rehearsal or class that require abrupt changes in direction can overstress the peroneal tendons. The patient will typically have pain and/or swelling posterior to the lateral malleolus.

PE On examination, the patient will likely have tenderness to palpation and/or swelling posterior to the lateral malleolus. Resisted ankle plantar-flexion and subtalar eversion may be painful. Passive ankle dorsiflexion and subtalar inversion may be painful.

Imaging/Diagnostic Evaluation An MRI may be helpful to evaluate bony or soft tissue pathology as well as the presence of tendon tears, and possible peroneal tendon subluxation.

Treatment For acute tenosynovitis symptoms, **PRICE** forms the mainstay of treatment. NSAIDs may be necessary for pain control initially. Immobilization in a short walking boot for 2–4 weeks may be necessary for severe symptoms. For milder symptoms, a lateral heel wedge, ankle brace, or arch support may help. In the acute phase, heat, ice, and ultrasound can reduce pain and swelling. A specific functional rehabilitation program that focuses on modalities, strengthening, and stretching is essential.

Surgical intervention is rarely required. This may include peroneal tenosynovectomy and tendon repair. Chronic peroneal tendon subluxation is more commonly associated with the need for surgical intervention. This may include various deepening procedures for the peroneal tendon groove in the lateral malleolus as well as repair of the peroneal retinaculum.

References

1. O'Kane JW, Kadel N. Anterior impingement syndrome in dancers. Curr Rev Musc Med 2008; 1(1): 12–16.
2. Nihal A., Rose D., Trepman E. Arthroscopic treatment of anterior ankle impingement syndrome in dancers. Foot Ankle Int 2005; 26(11): 908–12.
3. Hamilton WG, Geppert MJ, Thompson FM. Pain in the posterior aspect of the ankle in dancers. Differential diagnosis and operative treatment. J Bone Joint Surg 1996; 78-A(10): 1491–1500.
4. Fernandez-Palazzi F, Rivas S, Mujica P. Achilles tendonitis in ballet dancers. Clin Ortho 1990; 257: 257–61.
5. Thermann H. Treatment of Achilles tendon ruptures. Foot Ankle Clin N Am 1999; 4: 773–87.
6. Maffulli N. Rupture of the Achilles tendon. J Bone Joint Surg Am 1999; 81: 1019–36.
7. Jozsa L, Kvist M, Balint BJ et al. Role of recreational sport activity in Achilles tendon rupture: a clinical, pathoanatomical and sociological study of 292 cases. Am J Sports Med 1989; 17: 338–43.
8. Hamilton WG. Sprained ankles in ballet dancers. Foot Ankle Int 1982; 3(2): 99–102.
9. Young CC, Niedfeldt MW, Morris GA, Eerkes KJ. Clinical examination of the foot and ankle. Prim Care: Clin Off Pract 2005; 32(1): 105–32.
10. Hamilton WG, Thompson FM, Snow SW. The modified Brostrøm procedure for lateral ankle instability. Foot Ankle Int 1993; 14(1): 1–7.
11. Noffsinger MA. Sever disease. Emedicine 2004; http://www.emedicine.com/orthoped/TOPIC622.HTM
12. Johnson KA, Strom DE. Tibialis posterior tendon dysfunction. Clin Ortho 1989; 239: 196–206.
13. Hintermann B, Gachter A. The first metatarsal rise sign: a simple sensitive sign of tibialis posterior tendon dysfunction. Foot Ankle Int 1996; 17: 236–41.
14. McCormack AP, Varner KE, Marymont JV. Surgical treatment for posterior tibial tendonitis in young competitive athletes. Foot Ankle Int 2003; 24(7): 535–38.

3
Knee and Shin Injuries

Case Report A 13-year-old boy presents to your office complaining of knee pain that is intermittent and associated with episodes of swelling. Occasionally, he feels the knee "lock" and at these times the pain is worse. It takes several minutes before he can move his knee comfortably after a locking episode.

Diagnosis   Osteochondritis dissecans(OCD)

Epidemiology More common in young boys ages 11–13 years.

Pathophysiology Osteochondritis dissecans describes a condition in which a fragment of cartilage detaches from the joint surface. The fragment may separate partially or completely. It is thought to arise from multiple possible etiologies, including trauma or ischemia, or it may be idiopathic. In dancers, the repetitive strain of dance classes or rehearsal can lead to symptoms. A hereditary component has also been reported. Indirect or direct trauma to the posterolateral medial femoral condyle or recurrent impingement of the tibial spine on the lateral medial femoral condyle with tibial internal rotation can occur. The theory behind ischemia as a possible cause arises from studies of the vasculature to subchondral bone. Initially, reports suggested that subchondral bone vasculature provided insufficient anastomoses and would be at risk for causing ischemia to subchondral bone; however, recent studies have refuted this theory.

In the knee joint, the lateral aspect of the medial femoral condyle is most commonly affected, followed by the weight-bearing surfaces of the medial and lateral femoral condyles and the patella or anterior intercondylar groove. Four stages have been used to describe osteochondral lesions. The first stage involves compression of subchondral bone and the second involves a partially detached fragment of bone. The third stage involves complete fragment detachment within the underlying crater bed, whereas the fourth stage involves complete fragment detachment from the crater bed and is otherwise known as a loose body.

From: *Musculoskeletal Medicine*: *Essential Dance Medicine*
By A. Bracilović, DOI 10.1007/978-1-59745-546-6_3,
© Humana Press, a part of Springer Science+Business Media, LLC 2009

History   The patient will typically complain of intermittent pain, "aching," and swelling in the knee. The patient may also have pain or weakness with full knee extension. If the cartilage is a loose body, the patient may complain of the knee locking, catching, sticking, or giving way. The patient will typically have worse pain with tibial internal rotation.

PE   Full range of motion of the knee in extension will probably be limited and/or cause painful symptoms. The patient may have pain with passive external rotation of the tibia. A palpable lesion may be felt. Motor strength may be demonstrated with quadriceps weakness of the affected leg. If the OCD lesion is located on the medial femoral condyle, Wilson's test can be useful. This test involves passive flexion of the knee to 90 degrees followed by internal rotation of the tibia. The patient slowly extends the knee and pain is reproduced as the tibial spine compresses the OCD lesion on the medial femoral condyle at about 30 degrees of flexion (Figure 3-1). The pain should subside with external rotation and relief of tibial spine compression.

Imaging/Diagnostic Evaluation   Standard AP and lateral radiographs can reveal the presence of an osteochondral lesion as lucency in the articular epiphysis. A bone scan will reveal the amount of osseous uptake and reflects the likelihood of osteochondral fragment healing. With increasing uptake, osteoblastic activity increases and the lesion is more likely to heal. Serial scans may be used to follow the lesion and modify treatment options. MRI can demonstrate the degree of fragment detachment and/or displacement, the presence of loose bodies or fluid and the quality of the articular surfaces.

Treatment   Stage I lesions, especially in skeletally immature patients, should be expected to go on to complete healing with non-operative treatment. In dancers, protected weight bearing is recommended to allow healing. Return to activity is recommended once the patient has no reported symptoms, a normal physical examination and evidence of a healing lesion on radiograph or MRI. If the patient is still symptomatic after 3 months of initial conservative therapy or has **stage II-IV** lesions, especially in skeletally

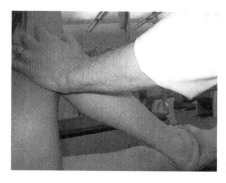

FIGURE 3-1. Wilson's test.

immature children, surgery should be considered. Also, in growing children whose physes are closing, surgery should be considered. Surgical options include arthroscopic subchondral drilling, debridement, fragment stabilization, excision, and open removal of loose bodies. Transplants of autologous chondrocytes with removal of sclerotic bone, excision of the defect and bone grafting are used when other treatment options have failed.

Case Report   An 18-year-old female modern dancer who is also a marathon runner presents to your office complaining of pain in front of one or both of her legs, which becomes worse in class after jumps and while running.

Diagnosis   Tibial stress syndrome, periostitis

Epidemiology   More common in dancers who rehearse on hard, uneven surfaces.

Pathophysiology   Several theories exist regarding the actual pathology causing medial and anterior tibial stress syndrome. They are normally assumed to involve inflammation of the periosteal sheath lining the tibia. Pain results from irritation of the periosteal sheath and/or the surrounding muscles and tendons. Periostitis typically occurs as an overuse injury associated with repetitive, forceful activities such as running and jumping. Recurrent overuse in rehearsals where the same sequence of movements is frequently repeated can lead to increased stress over the tibia. Repetitive forced ankle dorsiflexion with increased weight bearing can cause a stress reaction. If left untreated, tibial stress syndrome can lead to stress fractures. The component of muscle fatigue is an important contributing factor, as the stress will be transferred to the bone once the muscles are sufficiently expended.

History   The patient will typically describe pain over the anterior or medial aspect of the tibia, worse following class and any jumping or running activity. Dancers who overpronate and have tight gastrocnemius and soleus muscles more frequently complain of periostitis or tibial stress reaction. The pain may vary in intensity and is usually located on the medial aspect of the tibia. The pain will usually persist for some time despite stopping class, rehearsal or other activity, and removing weight bearing. It is also always important to suspect the female athlete triad when evaluating dancers for stress reactions or stress fractures.

PE   Palpation of the medial tibia over the middle to lower third of the bone will typically be tender in adults, and in children tenderness over the anterior proximal one third of the tibia is more common. It is also important to examine the patient's gait and observe biomechanical imbalances in walking, *plié*, and *relevé*. The patient's street shoes as well as dance shoes should be inspected for signs of wear and hyperpronation. Chronic exertional anterior compartment syndrome should be **differentiated** by lack of tightness and discomfort localized to the anterior compartment musculature (tibialis anterior), especially with repetitive resisted ankle dorsiflexion.

Imaging/Diagnostic Evaluation   Radiographs are typically normal; however, should always be obtained if a stress fracture is suspected. A bone scan is most sensitive to diagnose a stress fracture and should be normal in a patient with only periostitis.

Treatment **PRICE** forms the initial mainstay of therapy. Dancers should initially reduce the amount of jumping and leaping in class while they are symptomatic and should especially try to avoid jumping on hard or uneven surfaces that lack the typical reinforcement of dance floors. NSAIDs may be helpful in controlling the pain acutely. Custom molded orthotics can be used to help correct hyperpronation for improved biomechanical alignment. A functional rehabilitation program focused on stretching the gastrocnemius, soleus muscles, and the Achilles tendon and strengthening the anterior tibialis and arch of the foot is essential. Gradual increase in activity is recommended over a 6-week period. The dancer should return to class and stage only when she or he no longer experiences pain with all dance activities. If chronic exertional anterior compartment syndrome is diagnosed and conservative management is not successful, a surgical release (decompression fasciotomy) is highly successful in treating the underlying condition.

Case Report   A 22-year-old female principal ballet dancer who smokes, has an eating disorder, and has not menstruated in the last 6 months presents to your office complaining of localized pain over the anterior aspect of her left shin, which becomes worse after rehearsal involving jumps and *grand jeté* (leaps) (Figure 3-2). She has also noticed a small, hard bump over the tender area. The pain occasionally bothers her at night.

Diagnosis   Tibial stress fracture

Epidemiology   Common type of stress fracture in dancers, typically overuse injury from jumping and running.

Pathophysiology   Stress fracture occurs often as the end result of a continuum—stress reaction followed by stress fracture. The anterior tibia is under tension and is prone to develop delayed or non-union. The anterior tibia is unable to handle the repetitive load on the bone without being given sufficient time to recover. Given dancers' demanding choreography, routines, and schedules, they are a perfect set-up for stress fractures to occur. The initial stress onto the bone may not be suspected as the patient may or may not feel pain; however, over time, the repeated submaximal load without adequate recovery forms a chronic cycle that eventually results in injury. Patients with a stress reaction typically have positive imaging findings without associated pain symptoms.

Physiologic risk factors associated with the development of stress fractures include disordered eating patterns, often seen in a dancer's restricted diet to maintain low weight, eating disorders, muscle weakness, and chronic amenorrhea. The female athlete triad of amenorrhea, disordered eating, and osteoporosis reflects an underlying estrogen deficiency and places the dancer at increased risk for the development of stress fractures. Smoking, excessive thinness, and hormonal deficiencies are often associated risk factors with dancers and further predispose them to injury.

History   A stress fracture is a clinical diagnosis and the patient's symptoms must correlate with radiographic findings. When suspecting tibial stress fractures or stress fractures in general, it is important to ask about prior injuries, physiologic risk factors such as amenorrhea, disordered eating and/ or eating disorders, as well as environmental risk factors, such as learning

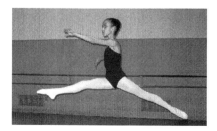

FIGURE 3-2. *Grand jeté.*

new choreography, rehearsing on a hard surface that is not an appropriately reinforced sprung dance floor or recently increasing amount of hours dancing. The patient will often report insidious onset of symptoms. The patient may have well localized or poorly localized pain, usually with jumps and *grand jeté* (leaps). In thin female dancers, insufficient amounts of estrogen are associated with loss of bone mineral density. This also predisposes them to stress fracture. Multiple studies have shown that amenorrheic and oligomenorrheic athletes are at higher risk for bone loss and that female runners with decreased bone mineral density are at higher risk for stress fracture [1]. It is important to obtain a full menstrual history when considering a diagnosis of stress fracture in young female dancers.

PE   Usually, the patient will have **localized bony tenderness** with a palpable protrusion over the anterior surface of the tibia. This is in contrast to the diffuse pain typically felt with periostitis. There may be associated warmth, erythema, and brawny edema.

Imaging/Diagnostic Evaluation   For stress fractures, plain radiographs will typically be initially negative. They can reveal evidence of a chronic stress fracture after 2–3 weeks. The "dreaded black line" best seen on lateral radiographs is typically described as a "horizontal fissure with adjacent hyperostosis" [2]. On AP radiographs, cortical thickening can be evident with widening of the anterior cortex, known as "buttressing" [2]. A bone scan is sensitive but not specific and can demonstrate the presence of a stress fracture more than 48 hours after symptoms begin and stay positive for up to 10 months. MRI is sensitive for stress fractures and will demonstrate decreased signal on T1 images with or without associated muscle or periosteal edema when a stress fracture is present. With chronic stress fractures, MRI will demonstrate increased signal in the anterior cortex of the tibia and may reveal altered integrity of the surface of the anterior tibial margin. In a stress reaction, MRI will typically reveal marrow edema and the bone scan will have minimal uptake.

Treatment   Whereas patients with a stress reaction should be instructed to reduce their dance activity, patients with anterior tibial stress fractures must **avoid** dance activity for 6–8 weeks. Early stress fractures should be treated with decreased axial loading and may require crutches for partial or non-weight bearing, depending upon severity of symptoms. Electropulsed electromagnetic field bone stimulation and low intensity–pulsed ultrasound are helpful. A functional rehabilitation program should focus on stretching of the gastrocnemius and soleus muscles and strengthening of the anterior tibialis muscle as well as the quadriceps and hamstrings. Hyperpronation and biomechanical alignment should be addressed and custom molded orthotics used as necessary. For patients with documented leg-length discrepancies, it is also important to address postural alignment issues and proper biomechanics to avoid recurrence of injury. NSAIDs should typically be avoided as they mask the patient's pain symptoms. The dancer should anticipate return to stage and rehearsal full-time approximately 6–8 months following injury. For stress fractures, it is essential to allow the bone time to heal. This is likely difficult for dancers to hear and adhere to; however, it is crucial that they rest in the short term to avoid further progression of their injury in the long term.

Treatment of the female athlete triad is also essential. This consists of nutritional and lifestyle counseling as well as hormonal replacement therapy. It is important to have a thorough discussion with the female dancer regarding her eating habits, the requirements of her dance schedule, and the importance of a healthy diet in preventing future injuries and the development of osteoporosis.

If the stress fracture does not show signs of healing after 6–8 months, surgery should be considered. Surgical options include drilling under fluoroscopic guidance, autogenous bone grafting, and occasionally these fractures may progress to complete fractures of the tibia, requiring intramedullary nailing [3].

Case Report   A 25-year-old Indian female *Bharatanatyam* dancer presents to your office complaining of anterior knee pain that has been worsening over the past 6 months. She states the pain is worse after holding the *Ardhamandala* (Figure 3-3) position throughout an entire dance performance. She also complains of difficulty holding the *Mandi* (Figure 3-4) position while doing a *Sabdam* item.

Diagnosis   **Anterior interval knee pain (AIKP), patellofemoral pain**

Epidemiology   Frequent cause of knee complaints in female dancers.

Pathophysiology   Several theories have been proposed to explain the specific underlying processes leading to AIKP. It is generally accepted to be multifactorial, involving mechanical and chemical changes in the patellofemoral joint. As the patella articulates with the patellofemoral groove in the femur, it rotates and tilts as well as moves superiorly, inferiorly, medially and laterally, with multiple resultant forces acting on the different points of contact between the undersurface of the patella and the femur.

  In Indian forms of dance such as *Bharatanatyam*, maintenance of a half seated, squatting position (*Ardhamandala*) is required for the duration of the piece and may also at times require the fully seated position (*Mandi*). Constant knee flexion increases the stress placed on the patella and, consequently, patellofemoral pain is a frequent complaint among *Bharatanatyam* dancers.

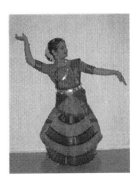

FIGURE 3-3. *Ardhamandala* position.

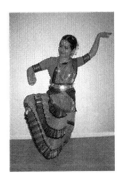

FIGURE 3-4. *Mandi* position.

In ballet dancers, the demand of frequent knee flexion combined with external rotation predisposes the dancer to excessive tibial torsion at the knee. Often, inadequate femoral retroversion at the hips and pronation at the subtalar joint, usually associated with *pes planus* or flat feet, result in disturbance of the normal patellofemoral alignment. The patella is pulled laterally, placing increased stress on the articular surfaces and lateral aspect of the patella. Over time, this increased wear in combination with poor technique and alignment can lead to clinical symptoms. Imbalance of the quadriceps muscles with miscoordinated firing of the lateral and medial quadriceps as well as a tight lateral retinaculum can also lead to abnormal tracking of the patella.

Dancers who have poor core control and are unable to maintain pelvic stability will tend to have increased anterior pelvic tilt, associated with femoral internal rotation and decreased recruitment of their hamstring muscles. In turn, loss of appropriate hip extension and gluteal and hamstring control leads to loss of control of tibial internal and external rotation. This subsequently leads to patellar instability, misalignment of the patella in the trochlear groove and can be associated with symptoms of knee pain.

Correct knee and ankle alignment in *plié* involves the patella aligning vertically over the first to third toes (Figures 3-5). *Plié* with the knee moving further anteriorly often reflects inadequate external rotation at the hips,

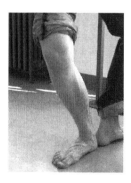

FIGURE 3-5. **(A)** Proper knee and ankle alignment.

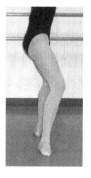

FIGURE 3-5. **(B)** Improper knee and ankle alignment.

resulting in an attempt to force external rotation from the tibia on the femur, which in turn places increased tensile stress on the medial aspect of the knee.

History   Patients with AIKP will most often present complaining of pain in *plié* positions. They will typically have anterior knee pain worse with ascending stairs, sitting with the knee flexed for a prolonged period of time or while running. The pain is typically of gradual onset and progression, diffuse in nature and may be associated with a sensation of the knee catching, giving way or feeling stiff.

PE   Tenderness can be elicited over the anterior aspect of the knee and may be diffuse or localized to the retropatellar surface. The "theater" sign reflects pain in the anterior knee after sitting for a prolonged period of time, as while watching a film in the theater. The Q angle refers to the angle formed between the line drawn from the anterior superior iliac spine through the central patella and the line drawn from the central patella to the tibial tubercle. Normally, this angle is approximately 8–13 degrees in males and 15–18 degrees in females [4]. Patellofemoral malalignment may be contributory to patellofemoral syndrome.

The J sign may be elicited when the patient flexes the knee to 30 degrees, with the patella abruptly shifting medially as it enters the trochlear groove. Others have described the J sign with extension of the knee from the seated position to zero degrees, with a positive J sign observed when the patella lateralizes in extension into an inverted J sign. A positive J sign has been reported to reflect either a tight lateral retinaculum, patellar instability or vastus medialis obliquus weakness, with subsequent increased lateral pull of the patella when contracting the quadriceps. When assessing the dancer's alignment, it is also important to assess the flexibility of the gastrocnemius muscles, the depth of *plié*, and the degree of tibial internal rotation and subtalar joint pronation.

Imaging/Diagnostic Evaluation   If a patient shows no improvement in 6 weeks following a prescribed treatment regimen, radiographs and possible MRI are recommended.

Treatment   Initially, **PRICE** and a course of individualized physical therapy based on establishing proper biomechanical alignment are essential, as AIKP is a multifactorial problem. The goal is to obtain core (abdominal and pelvic) as well as lower extremity strength and flexibility, which will lead to greater control of movement as well as correct biomechanics. Therapy should include exercises for strengthening the hip abductors, gluteal muscles, quadriceps as well as iliotibial band, hamstring, and calf stretching. Closed kinetic chain exercises are generally recommended as they place less stress on the knee joint than full arc isotonic exercises. However, open chain exercises from 25 to 90 degrees are useful to reenact common and, usually, necessary movements of daily activity, including walking, negotiating stairs, etc. Relative rest is recommended for the component of patellofemoral pain that is often associated with overuse and overload. In dancers, it is essential to correct underlying faulty technique, including the attempt to force turnout from the knees and feet instead of using the deep external rotators of the hip.

While performing the Indian dance *Bharatanatyam*, dancers should ensure placement of the feet completely on the ground with the heels down in the *Ardhamandala* position. Swaying of the waist and bending forward with increased lumbar flexion should be avoided. When tapping the feet, correct *Ardhamandala* posture should be maintained without straightening of the legs.

Patients who incorporate running in their exercise regimen may change to lower impact activity such as running on an elliptical machine, spinning, stationary biking, or swimming. Use of a neoprene knee sleeve or knee brace is controversial and probably more appropriate for significantly lateral patellar subluxation. Footwear that fits appropriately as well as arch supports or custom orthotics may help improve the biomechanics of the lower extremity in maintaining a stable base of support for a normal, *pes planus* or *pes cavus* foot.

Often, surgery is indicated only if non-operative management has been unsuccessful for a period of 6 months to a year. Degenerative cartilage behind the patella and/or impinging hypertrophic synovitis can be removed arthroscopically. If the patient's pathology is characterized by significant lateral patellar tracking that is not improved with stretching of the iliotibial band or strengthening of the quadriceps, release of the lateral retinaculum may help [5]. For patellofemoral malalignment recalcitrant to the above, a tibial tubercle transposition may be required to correct the malalignment, although this is avoided if at all possible in dancers.

Case Report   During a performance for which you are the physician on call, a 34-year-old male ballet dancer collapses on stage following a single leg landing from a hitchkick with subsequent buckling of his right knee. Backstage, he tells you that he felt and heard a "pop" in his knee as well as immediate pain and swelling.

Diagnosis   Anterior cruciate ligament rupture

Epidemiology   Low incidence among elite ballet and modern dancers. Three-to-five times greater relative risk in female modern dancers than female ballet dancers and male dancers, most commonly via single leg landing from jumps [6].

Pathophysiology   Injuries to the ACL result from a decelerative force on the knee, often combined with a rapid change in the direction of movement. In dance, ACL injuries and tears are often associated with landings from jumps, when the dancer is pivoting, side-stepping, or turning sharply. Landing on a single leg from a jump has been shown to result in increased internal rotation of the knee, increased knee valgus at 40 degrees of knee flexion, decreased knee flexion upon landing, and increased vertical ground reaction force. Further studies have shown support for the theory of ligament dominance to explain the etiology of ACL injuries in dancers, with the finding that women land more often with increased knee valgus when compared to men [7]. Hyperlaxity and increased tibial torsion as measured by an increased thigh-foot progression angle have also been cited as risk factors for ACL injury [8]. The remaining number of injuries usually occurs via direct contact and results in injury to multiple surrounding ligaments in the knee, including the lateral collateral ligament or medial collateral ligament.

History   The patient will typically complain of the knee giving way upon landing from a jump or twisting the knee sharply. The knee may feel unstable, insecure, or as if it is hyperextended. Pain is typically associated with feeling and hearing a "pop," as well as decreased range of motion and swelling. Depending on the activity, the patient may or may not be able to continue.

PE   Acutely, the patient will typically have decreased range of motion of the affected knee. Often, a knee effusion is present secondary to the ACL has been compromised. Joint line tenderness may occur if associated bone bruising or meniscal tears are present. Tests for ligament instability, including Lachman and the anterior drawer tests, should be performed on both knees for comparison. To perform the Lachman test, hold the knee in 20–30 degrees of flexion while stabilizing the patient's femur in one hand and proximal tibia in the other (Figure 3-6). The test is positive when there is increased excursion and no distinct endpoint of tibial excursion. The anterior drawer test involves placing the patient's knee in 90 degrees of flexion while stabilizing the foot flat on the table (Figure 3-7). The proximal tibia is

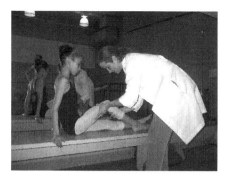

FIGURE 3-6. Lachman test.

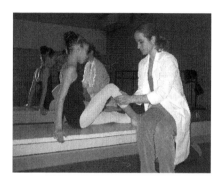

FIGURE 3-7. Anterior drawer test.

pulled anteriorly toward the examiner while holding the proximal calf in both hands, fingers over the insertion of the hamstrings, and thumbs over the lateral and medial joint lines. Lack of a firm endpoint with increased excursion of the tibia compared to the unaffected side may also indicate an ACL tear, although this maneuver is considered less sensitive than the Lachman test.

Imaging/Diagnostic Evaluation   Standard AP and lateral radiographs should be obtained to rule out fracture or dislocation, and can reveal an avulsed piece of bone from the lateral tibia, known as a Segond fracture. MRI is helpful to demonstrate a torn ACL as well as associated injury, including meniscal tears, femoral or tibial bruising, and edema.

Treatment   Depending on the age of the patient, level of dance activity (amateur to professional) and any associated injury, treatment of an acute ACL tear can vary. If there are associated injuries in addition to the ACL tear, surgery and aspiration of a painful hemarthrosis may be required. Initial pre-operative and post-operative rehabilitation programs are similar. Acutely post injury, **PRICE** is recommended to reduce pain and inflammation. A functional rehabilitation program focusing on restoration of range of motion and strength is essential. Although non-operative management may yield a potentially faster return to dance activity, studies have shown that more than 80% of dancers will require **ACL reconstruction** to be able to return to full, unrestricted dance activity [9]. In elite dancers who require maximal knee stability and restoration of full range of motion, arthroscopic reconstruction of the ACL is usually recommended. The technique of arthroscopic reconstruction of the ACL continues to evolve, with grafts made from autogenous patellar tendon, quadruple strand hamstrings (semi-tendinosus and gracilis), quadriceps tendon, allograft, and synthetic ligaments. One survey of multiple techniques for ACL reconstruction showed 92% of dancers returning to dance activity without restrictions, 6% modifying their dance technique to avoid jumps and 2% opting to choose another career [10].

Post-operatively, rehabilitation starts early with quadriceps co-contractions and partial weight bearing. A knee immobilizer with crutches and progressive partial weight bearing are typically recommended post-operatively for 5 days and full weight bearing as tolerated is started 5 days post-operatively. Functional rehabilitation should focus on progressive resistance exercise to improve muscular strength, control excessive tibial translation, and achieve dynamic stabilization. Hamstring isotonic and closed chain quadriceps strengthening exercises are recommended as soon as the patient is able to tolerate. Patients can typically return to full dance activity by 6 months following surgery.

Case Report   A 29-year-old male ballet dancer presents to your office complaining of anterior knee pain that is worse after allegro combinations, especially with landing from jumps. He does not recall a specific time of onset or any instigating injury. The pain occasionally resolves during class, but recently has persisted after finishing class or rehearsal.

Diagnosis   Patellar tendonitis

Epidemiology   Also known as jumper's knee.

Pathophysiology   During jumping and specifically upon landing, the patellar tendon is placed under significant stress from the eccentric contraction of the quadriceps muscles. Landing from a jump has a net downward force; however, the quadriceps contract eccentrically in the opposite direction to decelerate and control the landing. When the knee is flexed, the patellar tendon sustains the greatest degree of stress at its insertion site. In dancers, the combination of tight quadriceps and hamstrings with poor landing technique exacerbates the load placed on the patellar tendon. Over time, the patellar tendon can develop chronic inflammatory and degenerative changes from repetitive microtrauma. Histologically, inflammatory cells are not usually a component of chronic patellar tendinopathy; therefore, patellar tendonitis is described in the acute phase.

History   The patient will typically present complaining of gradual onset of anterior knee pain without specific time of onset or preceding injury. The pain is typically aching, dull, worse with landing from jumps, and located inferior to the patella.

PE   On exam, the patient will usually have full active range of knee motion; however, usually has decreased quadriceps excursion. There may be point tenderness inferior to the patella. Pain is elicited with resisted terminal knee extension, from 30 to 0 degrees. If pain is superior to the patella, consider insertional quadriceps tendonitis. Patellar tendonitis has been previously classified into 4 stages. **Stage I** involves pain following activity, without affecting performance. Pain in the first stage resolves with rest. **Stage II** involves pain during and following activity, without affecting performance. The pain may resolve following warm-up, but returns after finishing the activity. **Stage III** involves pain during and following activity and affects the quality of performance. **Stage IV** involves pain, inability to completely extend the knee, a sensation of the knee "giving way" and may reflect a partial tear of the tendon.

Imaging/Diagnostic Evaluation   Standard radiographs may reveal a small contributory inferior patellar osteophyte in the symptomatic region, which is usually unremarkable. Ultrasound and MRI can demonstrate specific tendon abnormalities. More recently, ultrasound with power Doppler has been used as a technique to localize neovascularized areas surrounding the patellar tendon.

Treatment First, patients should be instructed to decrease the dance activity that aggravates the pain and increases the load placed on the patellar tendon, typically small and large jumps. **PRICE** is important initially, followed by an individualized functional rehabilitation program. Cryotherapy and ultrasound can be used initially with **stage I** injuries. Oral anti-inflammatories may be useful in the acute phase to reduce pain. Stretching of the quadriceps is essential. Strengthening of the quadriceps starting with closed chain exercises emphasizing the eccentric phase on a decline board is recommended [11, 12]. Stretching should be in the painless range of motion, usually from 90 to 30 degrees of flexion. Exercises should progress to plyometric exercises and include joint proprioceptive training. Patellar taping techniques are used to reduce friction on the patella and relieve pain. Custom molded orthotics can help reduce foot pronation, maintain a neutral subtalar joint position, and minimize excess tibial torsion forces that may be causing abnormal patellar tracking. In **stage III** of injury, a longer period of relative rest from inciting painful activity is recommended, for up to 6 weeks. During this time, an appropriate alternative strength-training and cardiovascular exercise program is important to prevent deconditioning.

In patients in whom conservative therapy has failed, ultrasound guided peritendinous corticosteroid and anesthetic injections have been reported to be effective [13], although if utilized, extreme caution should be exercised to avoid injecting directly into the patellar tendon for risk of tendon rupture. Surgical intervention for failed conservative therapy over an extended period of time or for **stage IV** injuries typically involves drilling and resection of the involved pole and partial debridement of the involved pathologic tendon.

Case Report   A 14-year-old male gymnast presents to your office complaining of anterior knee pain worse following class and rehearsal and after sitting or standing for a prolonged period of time. His knee "catches" occasionally, at which point the pain is worse, although he can fully range the knee in flexion and extension. He denies associated swelling or preceding injury.

Diagnosis   Plica syndrome

Epidemiology   Usually associated with pseudo-locking of the knee in dancers.

Pathophysiology   Synovial plicae (singular: plica, from the Latin meaning "fold") are remnants of fetal membranes that grow during embryonic development. Initially, the knee is divided into three separate components in the embryo. These membranes are typically resorbed by the second trimester; however, remnants that persist in adults are synovial folds and are termed plicae. They are typically characterized as four different types, depending on their location in the knee. These include the suprapatellar, infrapatellar, medial, and lateral plicae. In dancers, the medial plica is most often irritated and prone to injury. It is called the medial shelf plica from its orientation in the coronal plane, with a suprapatellar origin, oblique course, and insertion onto the infrapatellar fat pad. When the knee is flexed, the plica can get irritated with overuse or from direct trauma as it is most prominent in this position. It has also been suggested that the plica can become inflamed with repetitive flexion of the knee, where the plica acts as a bowstring, causing abrasion to the medial femoral condyle, although this theory is debated. Adjacent anterior synovial tissue or the infrapatellar fat pad may become hypertrophic, resulting in an anterior impingement syndrome as well.

History   The patient will typically complain of intermittent anteromedial or anterolateral knee pain that may be associated with clicking, catching, snapping, and/or occasionally giving way. Plica syndrome is typically associated with pseudo-locking, which involves clicking and catching as the patella moves within the femoral groove. True locking prevents the knee from further knee flexion or extension. The symptoms are worse during dance class or rehearsal, prolonged standing, sitting, squatting, or ascending stairs. It is important to ask about swelling of the knee, as plica syndrome typically does not cause swelling, in contrast to meniscal or ligamentous injuries.
Localized soft tissue swelling may occur, however, if there is associated synovial or fat pad impingement.

PE   Examination will typically reveal tenderness to palpation along the inferomedial patella, and it may be possible to palpate a tender, hypertrophied band. It is important to exclude associated meniscal or ligamentous injuries, patellar instability or tendonitis. Plica syndrome is typically not associated with an intra-articular effusion.

Imaging/Diagnostic Evaluation   Standard AP and lateral radiographs as well as MRI of the knee will help exclude other diagnoses; however, are usually not definitive for plica or synovial impingement syndrome. Plicae are often incidental findings during arthroscopic procedures and may or may not be symptomatic.

Treatment   Dancers are usually first instructed to use **PRICE** to relieve pain and inflammation. Physical therapy should focus on quadriceps, hamstrings, adductors, and gastrocnemius stretching as well as quadriceps and hamstrings strengthening exercises. The goal of therapy is proper patellofemoral alignment and specific technique modifications should be made to optimize the dancer's patellofemoral biomechanics in class. A neoprene knee sleeve may provide biofeedback and remind the dancer of proper alignment. A localized corticosteroid injection into the palpated plicae or inflamed synovium may help reduce inflammation. Further treatment options for failure of conservative management over an extended period of time include arthroscopic surgery to resect the plicae and/or inflamed synovium. Post-operatively, the patient follows a similar physical therapy program to restore full range of motion, appropriate quadriceps control and strength with gradual return to dance specific training. Good functional outcomes have been reported in patients treated with arthroscopic plica excision [14].

Case Report   A 17-year-old recreational ballet dancer presents to your office complaining of medial knee pain gradually worsening over the past few weeks. She notices the pain most during *grand pliés* and jumps. She also complains of the knee "locking up" on her from time to time, which is associated with excruciating pain.

Diagnosis   Meniscal tear

Epidemiology   Common injury in dancers as a result of increased flexion and torque at the knee joint.

Pathophysiology   The medial and lateral menisci are "C" shaped segments of fibrocartilage located between the tibial plateau and the femoral condyles. They act as shock absorbers to distribute the load transmitted through the knee joint during knee flexion and extension, and protect the femoral and tibial joint surfaces from excess friction. In ballet dancers, injuries to the meniscus may result from attempting to incorrectly increase turnout by placing the feet in the abducted first through fifth positions and straightening or "screwing" both knees. Acute injury to the meniscus is usually the result of direct trauma involving some type of rotational force. The dancer may land incorrectly from a jump with either a valgus (black arrow) or varus (white arrow) force applied to a flexed knee (Figures 3-8). A medial meniscal

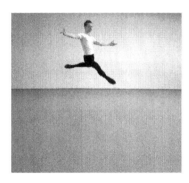

FIGURE 3-8. **(A)** Landing from a Bournonville jeté.

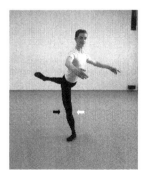

FIGURE 3-8. **(B)** Mechanism of injury: valgus and varus stresses.

tear can result from a valgus force applied to an internally rotated femur with the foot grounded and knee flexed. A lateral meniscal tear can occur with a varus force applied to an externally rotated femur with the knee hyperflexed. In *plié*, when landing from jumps and when squatting with the knee hyperflexed, as in specific types of folk dancing, the lateral meniscus is at higher risk for injury.

History   The patient will typically complain of pain over the medial or lateral joint line, associated with inability to completely extend or flex the knee. If the tear occurs through the vascular outer third of the meniscus, swelling can develop from hemarthrosis. The patient may also complain of the knee locking or buckling, which reflects a fragment of torn cartilage that can lodge in the joint, limiting extension or causing pain. This type of buckling should be distinguished from that caused by joint instability as seen in ligamentous injuries or reflex inhibition of the quadriceps due to pain. If the tear is minor, the patient may initially not notice pain until some time has passed and further activity frays the torn cartilage.

PE   Examination will typically reveal decreased range of motion and joint line tenderness to palpation over the involved medial or lateral side. Inspection may reveal atrophy of the quadriceps muscles if the injury is more than a week old. Pain can be elicited with hyperflexion of the knee or with deep squatting when the posterior horn of the medial meniscus is involved. In the dancer, the pain may be reproduced with jumps, *plié*, or *développé*. There may be a knee effusion, although the presence or amount of effusion does not reflect the presence of a meniscal tear. Tests for ligamentous stability should be performed to rule out associated injuries (Figures 3-9 and 3-10).

To help localize meniscal involvement, a few provocative tests are useful: The McMurray test is performed with the patient supine and the hip and knee flexed. With the ankle in one hand, the tibia is externally rotated and a valgus force is applied to the knee. The knee is then extended, keeping the tibia externally rotated while applying a medial valgus force to the knee with the other hand (Figures 3-11). A palpable or audible click, pop, or snap reflects a

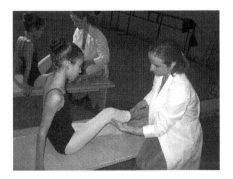

FIGURE 3-9. Test for medial collateral ligament laxity.

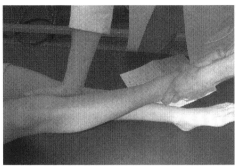

FIGURE 3-10. Test for lateral collateral ligament laxity.

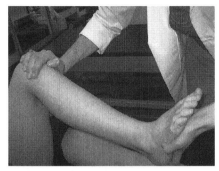

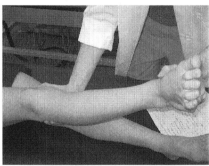

FIGURE 3-11. **(A, B)** McMurray test for medial meniscal tear.

likely tear of the posterior horn of the medial meniscus. McMurray test, however, is often not positive in the presence of a meniscal tear. The Apley compression test is performed with the patient lying prone with the affected knee flexed to 90 degrees. Holding the heel in one hand and stabilizing the knee in the other, a vertical downward force is applied through the knee and onto the menisci while rotating the tibia externally and internally. Pain with compression often reflects a meniscal tear (Figures 3-12). The Apley distraction test is useful to differentiate meniscal from ligamentous injury. In this test, the patient is placed in a position identical to the Apley compression

FIGURE 3-12. **(A, B)** Apley compression test.

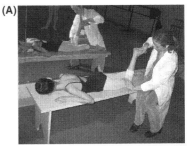

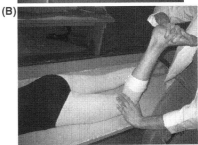

test and the tibia is externally and internally rotated; however, a vertical upward force is applied to the tibia (Figure 3-13). This maneuver relieves pressure off the menisci and reflects ligamentous injury if pain is elicited, i.e. medial or lateral collateral ligament sprain or tear.

Imaging/Diagnostic Evaluation   Radiographs are not helpful for the diagnosis of meniscal tears, although they may indicate associated degenerative knee pathology. MRI is the gold standard for accurate diagnosis of meniscal tears and will also demonstrate associated ligamentous, cartilage, and bony integrity.

FIGURE 3-13. Apley distraction test.

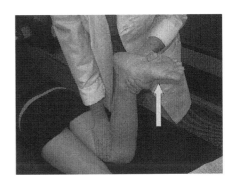

Treatment   Initially, **PRICE** helps reduce acute pain and inflammation. Non-steroidal anti-inflammatories help reduce swelling and pain. As the pain resolves, physical therapy focusing on restoration of range of motion and quadriceps strengthening should begin. Modification of dance activity should be individualized depending on the extent of the tear and physical demands of the patient's dance schedule. If the patient's pain and effusion improve over 4 to 6 weeks, gradual return to dance activity is recommended. Rarely, an intra-articular knee corticosteroid injection may be considered to reduce inflammation and pain. However, if pain, locking, or swelling persists, arthroscopic surgery should be considered.

Operative management of meniscal tears involves arthroscopic repair or excision of the meniscal tear. Care is taken to preserve as much viable cartilage as possible to avoid future injury, instability, and degenerative changes in the knee joint. Post-operative rehabilitation is similar to the course delineated above; however, initial restrictions are placed on the weight-bearing status to allow for wound healing. Gastrocnemius and soleus stretching exercises and ankle range of motion exercises are added to maintain functional range of motion prior to full weight bearing. Dancers are typically able to return to a full class and rehearsal schedule 6–8 weeks post-operatively. Meniscal repair, rather than excision of the meniscal tear, may require 6 weeks of non-weight bearing and as many as 6 months prior to return to full dance. Care must be exercised in the dancer if a repair is performed to avoid permanent post-operative restriction of range of motion due to capsular scarring.

References

1. Myburgh KH, Hutchins J, Fataar AB et al. Low bone mineral density is an etiologic factor for stress fractures in athletes. Ann Intern Med 1990; 113: 754–59.
2. Burrows HJ. Fatigue infraction of the middle of the tibia in ballet dancers. J Bone Joint Surg 1956; 38 B(1): 83–94.
3. Kadel NJ, Teitz CC, Kronmal RA. Stress fractures in ballet dancers. Am J Sports Med 1992; 20: 445–49.
4. Johnson LL, van Dyk GE, Green JR et al. Clinical assessment of asymptomatic knees: comparison of men and women. Arthroscopy 1998; 14: 347–59.
5. Juhn MS. Patellofemoral pain syndrome: A review and guidelines for treatment. Am Fam Physician 1999; 60 (7): 2012–22.
6. Liederbach M, Dilgen FE, Rose DJ. Incidence of anterior cruciate ligament injuries among elite ballet and modern dancers: A 5-year prospective study. Am J Sports Med 2008; 36(9):1779–1788.
7. Pappas E, Sheikhzadeh A, Hagins M et al. The effect of gender and fatigue on the biomechanics of bilateral landings from a jump: Peak values. J Sports Sci Med 2007; 6: 77–84.
8. Uhorchak JM, Scoville CR, Williams GN et al. Risk factors associated with noncontact injury of the anterior cruciate ligament: a prospective four-year evaluation of 859 West Point cadets. Am J Sports Med 2003; 31 (6): 831–42.
9. Cheung Y, Magee TH, Rosenberg ZS, Rose DJ. MRI of anterior cruciate ligament reconstruction. J Comp Assist Tomo 1992; 16: 134–37.

10. Chen L, Cooley V, Rosenberg T. ACL reconstruction with hamstring tendon. Ortho Clin N America 2003; 34 (1): 9–18.
11. Kongsgaard M, Aagaard P, Roikjaer S et al. Decline eccentric squats increases patellar tendon loading compared to standard eccentric squats. Clin Biomech 2006; 21 (7): 748–54.
12. Jonsson P, Alfredson H. Superior results with eccentric compared to concentric quadriceps training in patients with jumper's knee: a prospective randomized study. Br J Sports Med 2005; 39 (11): 847–50.
13. Fredberg U, Bolvig L. Significance of ultrasonographically detected asymptomatic tendinosis in the patellar and Achilles tendons of elite soccer players. Am J Sports Med 2002; 488–91.
14. Johnson DP, Eastwood DM, Witherow PJ. Symptomatic synovial plicae of the knee. J Bone Joint Surg Am 1993; 75 (10) 1485–96.

4
Hip Injuries

Case Report   A 50-year-old male artistic director of a professional ballet company presents to your office complaining of pain in both hips, left worse than right, which has been gradually worsening over the past 2–3 years. He has difficulty demonstrating certain movements in class and feels he has lost full range of motion in his hips.

Diagnosis   Osteoarthritis

Epidemiology   Can develop earlier in dancers than in the general population.

Pathophysiology   In dancers, osteoarthritis can be primary or secondary in origin. Primary arthritis refers to osteoarthritis without known etiology. Secondary arthritis can develop as a result of or following some type of injury. In dancers, repetitive microtrauma to the hip joints combined with improper biomechanics can lead to secondary arthritis. Osteoarthritis involves a degenerative process affecting the articular cartilage of the synovial joints, which include the hip, knee, and hand most often. Following repetitive microtrauma, small tears initially develop in the joint cartilage at the articular surface and ultimately progress to larger tears where the cartilage frays into smaller fragments.

In response to this cartilage damage, chondrocytes attempt to repair the joint surface and replenish the joint with new cartilage. However, the newly formed cartilage is not as strong as the original, may overgrow, and is more likely to tear again. Osteophytes are formed peripherally along the joint and the subchondral bone beneath the surface becomes sclerotic. Synoviocytes that normally produce hyaluronic acid that lubricates the healthy joint and provides necessary viscosity and elasticity cannot provide sufficient lubrication to the osteoarthritic joint, and water begins to replace the healthy synovial fluid. With further damage to the cartilage and loss of the

From: *Musculoskeletal Medicine*: *Essential Dance Medicine*
By A. Bracilović, DOI 10.1007/978-1-59745-546-6_4,
© Humana Press, a part of Springer Science+Business Media, LLC 2009

shock-absorbing, lubricating, and nourishing properties of healthy synovial fluid, the surrounding bone, ligaments, and tendons of the affected joint capsule bear the load of the joint and pain is felt.

The pain of osteoarthritis is believed to result from a number of different factors, as cartilage itself is not innervated. The pain can come from activation of nociceptive nerve endings in the surrounding synovium, bone, tendons, and ligaments that are placed under excess pressure. This leads to loss of the normal synovial cushion and cartilage lining. Pain can also result from vascular congestion of subchondral bone, periosteal elevation, muscle fatigue, and ultimately contracture of the joint.

History The patient will typically complain of pain that began gradually, with or without an inciting injury. The pain is worse with activity, relieved with rest, and associated with **morning stiffness lasting less than 30 minutes**.

PE Depending on the stage of disease, physical examination of the hip joint may differ. In the early stage, the patient may have antalgic gait, although the joint otherwise can appear normal. As the disease progresses, range of motion in the hip will become limited, with internal rotation typically affected before external rotation. Progressive hip flexion, adduction, and prone rotation are typically painful.

In ballet dancers, it is important to evaluate the alignment of the pelvis in common positions, such as *plié*, which is the beginning and endpoint for many exercises at the barre and in center. Correct *plié* technique involves activation of the external rotator muscles of the hips and adductor muscles of the legs, activating the adductors to work eccentrically when flexing the knees in *plié* and concentrically during knee extension (Figures 4-1).

Imaging/Diagnostic Evaluation Early in the disease process, standard radiographs are usually negative. As the disease progress, radiographs are useful to characterize the extent of disease. A universally accepted method of radiographically classifying arthritis is the Kellgren and Lawrence grading system, which identifies four characteristic radiographic features of arthritis [1]

1. Joint space narrowing
2. Osteophytes
3. Subchondral sclerosis
4. Subchondral cysts

Treatment It is important to inform the dancer that osteoarthritis is not an inevitable byproduct of aging and a lifetime of dancing. Rather, they should be made aware of several effective measures to manage the symptoms of osteoarthritis. First, changes in diet should be made to include adequate hydration (with water, not sugar filled drinks), increased intake of fruits, vegetables and cold-water fish, and decreased consumption of red meat and processed foods. Second, an individualized physical therapy program for

FIGURE 4-1. (**A**) *Demi plié* correct pelvic alignment.

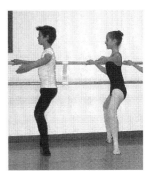

FIGURE 4-1. (**B**) *Demi plié* incorrect pelvic alignment.

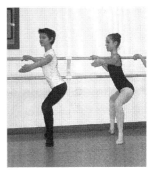

arthritis of the hip should focus on quadriceps and hamstring stretches, hip flexor and hip external rotator stretches, quadriceps, hamstrings and gluteal strengthening exercises and core strengthening exercises. Aerobic conditioning with low-impact weight-bearing exercises should also be emphasized.

Intra-articular injections of corticosteroid and sodium hyaluronate may be helpful in providing temporary pain relief [2]. Fluoroscopic guided corticosteroid injections have been reported to have anti-inflammatory and pain relieving effects for about 4–6 weeks. Due to possible cartilage damage, intra-articular steroid injections should be limited. Intra-articular injection of sodium hyaluronate for hip osteoarthritis using different types of hyaluronic acid formulations (Synvisc™, Hyalgan™, Supartz™, Orthovisc™, and Euflexxa™) have been used to provide pain relief and delay total hip arthroplasty, with variable results. Ultrasound guidance has been used with increasing frequency [3].

Indications for surgery typically include pain, functional limitations, and joint stiffness. In the dancer, surgical options for hip osteoarthritis include almost exclusively total hip arthroplasty. Osteotomy, arthrodesis, and hemiarthroplasty are not recommended. About 85% of patients undergoing total hip arthroplasty have the diagnosis of osteoarthritis. Hip arthroscopy has a limited role, if at all, in the management of osteoarthritis of the hip, with approximately 15% good to excellent results (D.J. Rose, personal communication).

Recently, newer techniques involving hip resurfacing have been used in younger patients. Whereas total hip replacement involves removal of the femoral head, hip resurfacing involves grinding down the head of the femur to a smaller ball and cementing a metal ball over the remaining head fragment to articulate with a new artificial metal socket. The advantages of hip resurfacing, however, over total hip replacement are at present debatable.

Case Report   A 20-year-old female modern dancer presents to your office complaining of pain over the right side of her hip that started gradually and is worse when sleeping on her right side, when ascending stairs and when standing up after sitting for a prolonged period of time.

Diagnosis   Trochanteric bursitis

Epidemiology   Common cause of hip pain in dancers, more common in females.

Pathophysiology   Trochanteric bursitis can develop acutely or gradually. It can occur from direct trauma to the hip, such as a fall. More often in dancers, it occurs as an overuse injury in combination with poor biomechanical alignment. Associated with trochanteric bursitis, the dancer may have a lumbosacral radiculopathy, scoliosis, snapping hip, or a leg length discrepancy. Trochanteric bursitis develops from inflammation of the bursa over the greater trochanter following repetitive stress to this area.

History   The patient can report localized pain over the greater trochanter that may be referred into the lateral thigh, less often to the posterior thigh or distal to the knee. It is typically worse with standing from a seated position, standing or walking for prolonged period of time, ascending stairs or sleeping on the affected side.

PE   Palpation of the affected greater trochanter will usually yield point tenderness. Active range of motion of the hip and lower back may be decreased, with pain reproduced in external rotation and abduction. The patient may have associated numbness or paresthesias in the proximal thigh that does not follow a specific dermatomal segment.

Imaging/Diagnostic Evaluation   Standard radiographs of the hip and femur can rule out associated fracture, dislocation, arthritis, bony, or soft tissue lesions. Radiographs may reveal trochanteric spur formation. Local injection of lidocaine into the trochanteric bursa may be diagnostic and therapeutic.

Treatment   Initially, a trial of oral NSAIDs may reduce pain and inflammation. A local corticosteroid injection into the bursa can also be therapeutic. In addition to medication, a course of physical therapy should be followed, focusing on stretching of the iliotibial band, tensor fascia latae, hip external rotators, hip flexors, and quadriceps. Ultrasound and TENS may also be helpful. Heel lifts may be prescribed for leg length discrepancy. For refractory trochanteric bursitis, arthroscopic or open bursectomy and trochanteric ostectomy may be surgical options.

Case Report   A 14-year-old female ballet dancer presents to your office complaining of an audible snapping sound as she brings her right leg into *passé développé à la seconde* (Figures 4-2). She denies any associated pain and cannot remember when exactly her hip started snapping, although she believes it has been over 2 years.

Diagnosis   *Coxa saltans*, **snapping hip syndrome**

Epidemiology   Very common among female ballet dancers younger than 20 years old.

Pathophysiology   *Coxa saltans*, otherwise known as the "snapping hip," has been classified into one of three sourcesexternal, internal, or intra-articular. External causes of snapping hip are thought to arise from the iliotibial band, tensor fasciae latae, or lateral margin of the gluteus maximus sliding over the greater trochanter. Internal snapping hip is very common in dancers and has been attributed to the iliopsoas tendon. Internal snapping hip has been attributed to the iliopsoas tendon sliding over the iliopectineal eminence, femoral head, femoral neck, or lesser trochanter. Internal snapping hip tends to be more painful than external, and may also be associated with iliopsoas bursitis or iliopsoas tendonitis involving inflammation of the synovium near the insertion of the tendon onto the femur. Intra-articular causes of a snapping hip have been attributed most often to loose bodies, labral tears, or osteochondral fracture. It has been suggested that repetitive hip flexion associated with snapping of the tendon can cause thickening and catching of the connective tissue band and may be associated with a tight

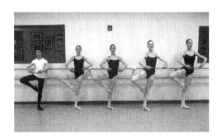

Figure 4-2. (**A**) *Passé.*

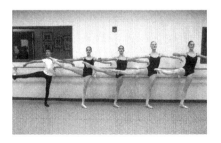

Figure 4-2. (**B**) *Passé développé à la seconde.*

iliotibial band, weak hip abductors, hip external rotators, poor core stability, and overpronation.

History The patient will typically complain of an audible snapping or clicking in the hip, particularly with *passé développé à la seconde* (involving flexion, abduction, and external rotation of the hip) and *grand plié* (Figures 4-3). The patient is usually able to voluntarily reproduce the snap, which is typically unilateral. There may be associated pain right before or during the snap but it is **often painless**. If associated pain is present, it may be felt laterally over the iliotibial band or gluteus maximus, or anteriorly in the groin over the iliopsoas. The snapping typically begins asymptomatically and can continue for months to years without causing pain.

PE Physical examination for a snapping hip may yield tenderness to palpation over the proximal iliotibial band, trochanteric bursa, or lateral gluteus maximus. The tenderness may be associated with an audible or palpable snap with *passé développé* actively. Flexion, abduction, and external rotation of the hip from a neutral position can typically elicit the snap. Weakness of the iliopsoas may be tested by resisted hip flexion in a turned out (externally rotated) position (Figure 4-4). *Coxa saltans* intra-articular, secondary to a labral tear, is associated with pain upon

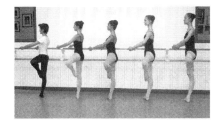

FIGURE 4-3. (**A**) *Passé* demonstrating hip external rotation.

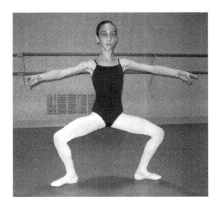

FIGURE 4-3. (**B**) *Grand plié.*

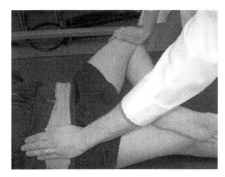

FIGURE 4-4. Resisted hip flexion.

passive forced flexion and adduction of the hip. However, this may also be positive with iliopsoas tendonitis, which can be ruled out by testing the iliopsoas. Therefore, this test should be considered sensitive for labral tears, but not specific.

Imaging/Diagnostic Evaluation   A snapping hip can typically be diagnosed from careful history and physical examination findings. Standard radiographs are typically normal and not recommended unless the diagnosis is uncertain. Ultrasound is helpful to visualize the anatomy and dynamic changes when moving the hip through flexion, abduction, and extension. Ultrasound is also useful to guide localized injection of the tendon sheath or bursa if iliopsoas tendonitis or bursitis is suspected. MRI/MRA is useful when assessing the etiology of snapping hip and when suspecting a labral tear. An intra-articular lidocaine injection may be utilized at the same time to differentiate intra-articular causes of anterior hip pain.

Treatment   For snapping hip syndrome that does not cause pain, treatment consists initially of correction of alignment, muscle imbalance and proper biomechanics and gait training. Anti-lordotic exercises, core strengthening exercises, lumbopelvic stability exercises, peripelvic stretching, and strengthening exercises should be emphasized. Hip flexor, hip abductor, and hip external rotator stretching exercises are important.

For an acutely painful snapping hip, **PRICE** and a short course of NSAIDs are usually appropriate. Physical therapy should focus on functional rehabilitation as above, as well as elimination of exacerbating dance activities until symptoms have resolved. For a snapping hip that is associated with iliopsoas tendonitis, please refer to the treatment of iliopsoas syndrome discussed in the next section. For *coxa saltans externa*, surgical options include resection of a portion of the iliotibial band overlying the greater trochanter or at the gluteus maximus insertion site and lengthening of the iliotibial band tendon. **Surgery in the dancer for a snapping hip should be avoided at all costs as this may end the dancer's career.**

Case Report   A 24-year-old female ballet dancer presents to your office complaining of painful snapping in the front of her hip when attempting *passé développé*and*attitude en avant* (Figures 4-5). It is worse after class and rehearsal and alleviated with rest.

Diagnosis   Iliopsoas tendonitis, iliopsoas syndrome

Epidemiology   Iliopsoas tendonitis, e.g. *coxa saltans interna*, is more common in student dancers than professional dancers.

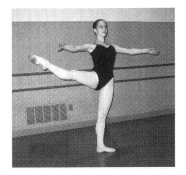

FIGURE 4-5. (**A**) *Développé* proper hip alignment.

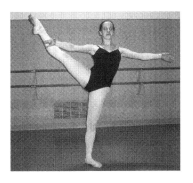

FIGURE 4-5. (**B**) *Développé* hip lifted.

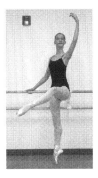

FIGURE 4-5. (**C**) *Attitude en avant* on pointe.

Pathophysiology In ballet dancers, the most common cause is overuse injury. Repetition of the basic *passé développé* preparation for many of the standard ballet positions involves hip flexion, abduction, and external rotation with extension of the leg to the maximum possible. Over time, repetition of these same movements leads to chronic microtrauma to the iliopsoas tendon. Without sufficient time to heal, microtrauma leads to macroscopic injury. Also, for young dancers, the adolescent growth spurt is a time of relative inflexibility of the hip flexors and hamstrings. Tight hip flexors exacerbate anterior pelvic tilt, placing the spine in excess lumbar lordosis with subsequent increased pressure on the posterior elements of the spine, leading to increased risk of back injury.

History The patient will typically complain of anterior hip pain that may be associated with clicking or weakness with *passé développé* (hip flexion, abduction, and external rotation). The pain is typically of insidious onset without acute preceding injury.

PE Physical examination will typically reveal tenderness to palpation of the iliopsoas in the femoral triangle, bordered superiorly by the inguinal ligament, laterally by the sartorius muscle and medially by the adductor longus muscle. The patient usually has tight hip flexors. Motor muscle testing usually reveals proximal weakness of the hip extensors and rotators. Provocative testing with active hip flexion in an externally rotated position can be applied with resistance with the patient lying supine. This is considered positive if anterior hip or groin pain is elicited with resisted active range of motion. Provocative hyperflexion of the hip is also painful when the patient's hip is gradually flexed while lying supine with the hip in neutral rotation and abduction [4]. If active and passive range of motion of the hip is normal, suspect iliopsoas tendonitis [5]. Anterior hip pain that occurs simply with passive range of motion and rotation of the hip with flexion, abduction, and adduction may be indicative of hip arthritis. If pain is felt posteriorly, suspect sacroiliac joint dysfunction. Forced flexion and adduction of the hip may be positive with both iliopsoas syndrome and labral tear.

Imaging/Diagnostic Evaluation Pelvic AP and frog leg lateral view radiographs will typically be normal, but are useful to rule out bony pathology. MRI is usually negative for iliopsoas pathology; however, may be useful to rule out other causes of anterior hip pain. Dynamic ultrasound can demonstrate tendinopathy, bursitis, edema, and other soft tissue pathology.

Treatment Acutely, the goal of treatment is to reduce pain and inflammation. **PRICE** is initially useful, followed by gentle stretching exercises once the symptoms have improved. For iliopsoas syndrome, iliopsoas and rectus femoris stretching and strengthening, as well as anti-lordotic and pelvic mobilization exercises should be instituted. This protocol has been found to resolve almost all instances of iliopsoas syndrome with the need for injection or surgery. Patients who overpronate can be helped by using a custom molded orthotic.

For patients with recalcitrant pain despite focused physical therapy and for whom iliopsoas tendonitis and/or bursitis is suspected, an ultrasound guided corticosteroid and local anesthetic injection into the iliopsoas tendon sheath or into the iliopsoas bursa may be beneficial. A lidocaine challenge test is performed under ultrasound guidance and involves bathing the iliopsoas tendon sheath with 1% lidocaine. If the patient experiences relief of his/her symptoms, the injection is both diagnostic and therapeutic. More recently, ultrasound guided peritendinous injections of a combination of corticosteroid and anesthetic have been used with increasing success in the treatment of tendonitis resistant to conventional therapy [6].

Almost all patients experience relief from symptoms with non-operative management. If conservative management is not successful over the course of 3–6 months, other causes of anterior hip pain should be explored. If, however, the above measures fail and the lidocaine injection challenge test does not relieve symptoms, surgical intervention may be considered. Surgical options include partial and complete release of the iliopsoas tendon and resection of the iliopsoas bursa via open and arthroscopic techniques; however, **surgery should absolutely be avoided in the active dancer as this may end his or her career**. In addition, operative complications have included persistent hip pain, weakness, and decreased sensation [7].

Case Report   A 20-year-old female modern dancer presents to your office complaining of low back pain and right buttock pain that is worse after rehearsals. She points with two fingers to her right lower buttock to a localizable area of pain.

Diagnosis   Sacroiliac joint dysfunction

Epidemiology   Accounts for 15% of chronic low back pain in general population [8] and approximately 12% of all dance injuries [9].

Pathophysiology   The sacroiliac (SI) joints articulate between the sacrum and the two ilia to provide significant stability as well as passive mobility. The sacroiliac articulation is unique in its role in relieving stress on the pelvic ring. It must allow movement of the pelvis secondary to significant range of motion of the lower extremities, especially in the extreme ranges displayed by dancers. On the other hand, it must also provide stability in absorbing forces transmitted from the spine into the lower extremities in multiple directions. The interlocking ridges and grooves joining the sacrum and two ilia as well as the surrounding ligaments allow this passive range of motion to occur.

In dancers, the SI joints are particularly stressed as the dancer transfers a significant amount of force through the torso into the lower extremities via the SI joints. These motions are also repetitive and the increased frequency and amount of force can ultimately lead to either asymmetric or decreased motion of these joints. The sacrum sits obliquely between the ilia, with its wider superior aspect tilting anteriorly. With hyperlordosis of the spine or exaggerated hyperextension of the spine or hip (Figure 4-6), the ilia tend to move anteriorly on the sacrum, with the wider superior portion of the sacrum moving inferiorly and the inferior portion moving superiorly. Both movements tend to separate the ilia and move them farther away from the sacrum. Decreased and asymmetric motion, which has been described and debated in various circles, can occur [10]. It is agreed that the sacroiliac joints respond to flexion, extension, and rotation of the trunk and lower limbs with complex gliding movements. Sacroiliac joint pain can occur as a

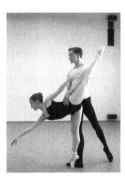

FIGURE 4-6. Hyperextension of hip in partnered *penché*.

result of acute injury to the surrounding ligaments, muscles, or nerves, or stress on the joints secondary to repetitive, extreme ranges of motion.

The innervation of the SI joints is purportedly broad, with multisegmental contribution from the dorsal rami of the L4, L5, S1, and S2 nerves, obturator nerve, superior gluteal nerve, and lumbosacral trunk. As a result, pain from this region can present with multiple referral pain patterns, including the buttocks, groin, thigh, and occasionally lower leg.

History The patient will typically complain of dull, aching pain in the buttocks, lower back, posterior thigh, groin, or occasionally lower leg. Dancers with sacroiliac joint hypermobility can also present with anterior hip pain. The pain may be worse with weight bearing and ipsilateral hip flexion and extension. The dancer may complain of decreased range of extension when performing maneuvers to the front and side and that the hip feels tight or locked. Assuming that the sacroiliac joint pain is secondary to biomechanical causes, it is still important to rule out other etiologies, including ankylosing spondylitis, other spondyloarthropathies, infection, and metabolic disease. Patients who are status post lumbar fusion, capsular tear, or subluxation may also have sacroiliac joint pain symptoms.

PE The patient may have gluteus medius weakness, tightness of the piriformis, or hip flexor muscles secondary to pain or muscle imbalance; however, strength, sensation, and reflexes should typically be normal. Palpation of the involved sacroiliac joint and surrounding soft tissue is usually painful. Provocative testing for sacroiliac joint dysfunction can be performed with the FABER or Patrick test, which involves flexion, abduction, and external rotation of the involved hip while applying pressure to the opposite anterior superior iliac spine (Figure 4-7). Gillet test is performed with the patient standing erect and alternating hip flexion while holding the knee to the chest as the examiner palpates the posterior superior iliac spines with both thumbs and observes for asymmetry of motion (Figure 4-8). Gaenslen test is performed by having the patient lie supine and flex the unaffected hip with the knee to the chest. The leg of the affected side is

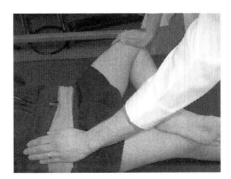

FIGURE 4-7. FABER test for sacroiliac joint dysfunction.

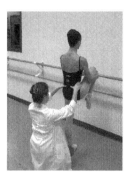

FIGURE 4-8. Gillet test.

dangled over the edge of the examining table with an inferiorly directed force applied to the leg to increase hip extension and load on the SI joint. SI joint provocative testing has not been shown to be reliably diagnostic or specific [11].

Imaging/Diagnostic Evaluation   Plain radiographs can demonstrate evidence of sacroiliac joint arthritis, which may or may not cause the patient symptoms. MRI is useful to demonstrate soft tissue pathology, sacral insufficiency fractures, inflammation, tumor, or abscess. Diagnosing the sacroiliac joint as the source of pain is best performed with intra-articular injections under fluoroscopic guidance. This method is preferred over radiographic evaluation or history of clinical symptoms and physical examination.

Treatment   PRICE, including anti-inflammatory medication, heat, and ice as needed are helpful for acute injury. Physical therapy is essential to correct improper technique and establish or reestablish proper biomechanics. Abdominal and hip abductor strengthening exercises as well as pelvic stabilization exercises are important. Avoidance of extreme ranges of motion in hip and lumbar spine hyperextension and flexion are recommended in the acute phase. Muscle spasm can be addressed with myofascial release and trigger point injections. A sacroiliac joint belt can provide proprioceptive awareness. Joint mobilization techniques and correction of any malalignment in positions at the barre or in center are important. If the above treatment measures do not significantly alleviate pain, consider an intra-articular anesthetic and steroid injection. Radiofrequency neurotomy has also been used with varying efficacy and involves ablation of the sacroiliac joint nerve branches.

Case Report A 40-year-old Pilates and yoga instructor who is also a secretary presents to your office complaining of pain in her right gluteal area after sitting in class or at her desk for a prolonged period of time. She is a smoker with a 25 pack-year history and admits to not warming up and stretching enough before or after class.

Diagnosis Piriformis syndrome

Epidemiology Occurs more commonly in females than males, although this syndrome is often overdiagnosed.

Pathophysiology The piriformis muscle is innervated by L5-S2 and passes through the greater sciatic notch to insert onto the superior surface of the greater trochanter. In hip extension, it externally rotates the hip, and in hip flexion, abducts the hip. Several anatomic variants have been observed of the course of the sciatic nerve in relation to the piriformis muscle. The sciatic nerve may pass undivided through the piriformis muscle or anterior to it. The piriformis muscle may be split by the peroneal portion of the sciatic nerve with the tibial portion passing anterior to the piriformis muscle. The peroneal portion may pass posterior to the piriformis with the tibial portion passing anterior to the muscle. Piriformis syndrome is often the result of some type of gluteal spasm, contracture, or trauma to the muscle that causes inflammation around the sciatic nerve. Gluteal spasm has been implicated in combination with tight hip flexors, sacroiliac hypomobility, and foot overpronation. This syndrome is often overdiagnosed, as it may be similar in presentation to other causes of pain in the gluteal region.

History The patient may complain of pain in the gluteal region, posterior thigh, calf and lateral foot, along the distribution of the sciatic nerve. The pain is typically of insidious onset and may be associated with low back pain, perineal pain, pain when rising from a seated position, defecating, or when sitting for a long period of time.

PE On physical examination, the patient will typically have tenderness to palpation in the gluteal region with pain with passive flexion, adduction, and internal rotation of the hip. The patient may have associated weakness with resisted hip external rotation and abduction. Lasègue sign reflects tenderness to palpation of the greater sciatic notch when the knee is extended with the hip flexed to 90 degrees. It is important to distinguish tenderness secondary to sciatic neuritis.

Imaging/Diagnostic Evaluation Electromyography (EMG) is useful to evaluate patterns of activity in specific muscles. In piriformis syndrome, the piriformis and gluteus maximus should show abnormal EMG activity, whereas the gluteus medius, gluteus minimus, and tensor fasciae latae should all be normal. An injection of lidocaine into the painful trigger point of the piriformis can be both diagnostic and therapeutic if the pain is relieved following injection.

Treatment   Dancers should avoid positions and activities that exacerbate the pain, such as prolonged sitting, bicycling, and repetitive *passé* positions in class or rehearsal. Therapeutic modalities including moist heat, cryotherapy, electrical stimulation, and ultrasound are beneficial prior to stretching exercises. Physical therapy should focus on stretching of the piriformis with flexion, adduction, and internal rotation of the hip (Figure 4-9). Stretching exercises should also involve the iliopsoas, gluteal muscles, tensor fasciae latae, and hamstrings. Myofascial release for tight lumbar paraspinal muscles and sacroiliac joint mobilization should be considered as needed. Heel lifts, yoga, soft tissue, and myofascial release techniques have also been recommended. More recently, injections of a mixture of corticosteroid and lidocaine as well as botulinum toxin into the piriformis muscle with either electromyographic, ultrasound, or fluoroscopic guidance have also been used. If the above non-operative interventions do not successfully alleviate the patient's symptoms, surgical options include release of the piriformis tendon near its insertion on the greater trochanter of the femur, resection of the piriformis muscle and sciatic neurolysis [12]. It is very important, however, to rule out other etiologies in the differential diagnosis prior to any invasive management.

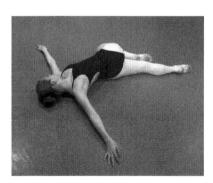

Figure 4-9. Piriformis stretch.

Case Report   A 28-year-old female principal ballet dancer presents to your office complaining of left groin pain that began approximately 6 months ago. She does not remember any acute injury and states the pain is worse during class and rehearsals. It occasionally bothers her at night. She thought the pain would resolve but it has persisted and now can get so bad that she has difficulty putting full weight on her leg.

Diagnosis   Femoral neck stress fracture

Epidemiology   Higher incidence in amenorrheic professional female dancers.

Pathophysiology   In dancers, frequent loading of the hip and femoral neck during class and rehearsal place high stresses with compressive and sheer forces on the relatively small femoral neck area. In ballet dancers, these stresses combined with low body fat, amenorrhea, and hypoestrogenemia greatly increase their risk of developing stress fractures. Without a necessary percentage of body fat, dancers' menstrual cycles stop, hypoestrogenemia develops, and their bones become weak and brittle. Initially, bone of the femoral neck can respond to the applied high stresses by increasing mechanical bone resorption, which is then balanced by osteoblastic bone remodeling. However, once the mechanical stresses combined with the metabolic hypoestrogenemia exceed the capacity of the bone to repair itself, microfractures develop that ultimately lead to fracture. A third pathophysiologic risk factor in dancers is poor technique as a result of muscle imbalance, further increasing the load placed on the femoral neck that should ideally be sustained by properly strengthened muscles.

History   The patient will typically complain of anterior hip, groin, or thigh pain that may refer to the medial knee via the obturator nerve. Typically, the pain has been going on for some time, may occur at night and be progressively worsening, or simply not resolving. The pain usually improves with rest and is worse with weight bearing and high impact activity. Often, the patient does not recall a specific initial injury.

PE   Depending on the severity of the fracture, the patient may or may not be able to bear weight on the leg. Tenderness to palpation of the femoral neck is actually not typical secondary to the soft tissue surrounding the femoral neck. Passive range of motion will typically be limited at end range. The patient may have pain with internal rotation of the hip and difficulty jumping on the affected leg. The patient should be assessed for leg length discrepancy and excessive subtalar pronation. Manual muscle testing may reveal weakness of the hip musculature, especially in hip flexion, which may be difficult to assess depending on the degree of pain.

Imaging/Diagnostic Evaluation   Initial radiographs are often not sensitive for fracture. A bone scan provides higher sensitivity and more information regarding any associated periosteal injury. MRI is important when considering surgical intervention and will demonstrate displacement of the fracture as well as associated soft tissue pathology.

Treatment   Depending on the location of the femoral neck stress fracture, management will vary. If the stress fracture is superolateral and is not displaced, it is considered a **tension** type fracture. Surgery (internal fixation) is usually required for non-displaced tension type femoral neck fractures as they are at high risk for displacement. If displacement occurs, the vascular supply to the femoral head may be compromised, which requires immediate surgery to avoid avascular necrosis.

Surgical intervention is also necessary for complete transverse femoral neck fractures and is typically performed via arthroplasty or internal fixation. It is important not to delay diagnosis of transverse femoral neck fractures for risk of non-union, malunion, delayed union, AVN, or osteonecrosis. Post-operatively, the patient usually begins toe touch weight bearing on days 2–3, followed with progressive weight bearing as tolerated with crutches, a walker, or other assistive aid for 8–12 weeks.

If the stress fracture is partial, occurring inferomedially, this is considered a **compression** type femoral neck fracture. Surgery is usually not indicated for this type of fracture as complete fractures and displacement tend not to occur. Weight bearing is initially avoided until the patient's pain symptoms improve, and subsequently should be limited to crutches or a cane in the hand opposite the injured side. Progressive weight bearing is allowed when pain free and healing of the fracture should be followed with serial radiographs. If after 3 months radiographs show fracture extension and/or the patient's symptoms are not improving, referral to an orthopedic surgeon is indicated.

Case Report   A 32-year-old professional female ballet dancer presents to your office complaining of sharp groin pain with hip flexion. The pain worsens by the end of class and following rehearsal. She also complains that her hip occasionally catches and gives way.

Diagnosis   Acetabular labrum tear

Epidemiology   Common cause of chronic hip pain in dancers secondary to repetitive stress at the extremes of hip range of motion and exacerbated by a hypermobile hip joint.

Pathophysiology   The acetabulum of the hip is covered by a fibrocartilaginous labrum similar to the glenoid labrum of the shoulder. The labrum provides joint stability by deepening the hip socket and reducing the stress on the hip joint. The acetabulum is oriented anteriorly and has the least amount of structural support in this direction. The stability of the capsule is largely provided by three ligaments—the iliofemoral ligament anteriorly, which is the strongest ligament in the body, the ischiofemoral ligament posteriorly, and the pubofemoral ligament inferiorly. Labral tears most commonly involve the anterolateral labrum.

In ballet dancers, it is important to remember that the degree of hip external rotation is dependent not only on the degree of femoral anteversion but also on the amount of tension provided by the iliofemoral ligament. As the hip externally rotates and extends, the femoral head glides anteriorly. Depending on the balance between tension and laxity of the ligaments forming the capsule as well as the depth of the hip socket itself, the relative mobility of the femoral head in the hip joint will vary. Excess capsular laxity can lead to instability, repetitive microtrauma from increased stresses on the hip joint, and eventually a labral tear. The increased stresses on the hip joint are usually associated with truncal rotation on a single weight bearing leg combined with hip external rotation, leg hyperabduction, and hyperextension of the spine.

In additional to lax ligaments, a large degree of external hip rotation can be secondary to shallow hip sockets, for which the body compensates with a large acetabular labrum. This will also lead to increased capsular laxity, instability, and potentially labral tears. In ballet dancers, it is further more difficult to distinguish labral tears as the cause or result of joint instability, as the requirement for hip external rotation must be balanced with adequate capsular support by the surrounding hip ligaments and musculature. The dancer ideally wants both a flexible and a well supported hip joint.

Risk factors for development of a labral tear include increased acetabular surface area due to acetabular bone spur formation (pincer impingement), increased femoral head radius or osteophyte formation (CAM impingement), acetabular retroversion, and hip dysplasia with a shallow acetabulum. The development of labral tears with associated hip joint instability, subluxation, and excessive joint loading has been associated with an increased risk of later developing degenerative hip osteoarthritis, which can ultimately necessitate hip replacement.

History   The patient can complain of anterior groin pain. Often the pain is sharp and associated with the sensation of the hip catching, clicking, giving way, or locking. The pain may be acute or chronic, depending on the mechanism of injury.

PE   For anterolabral tears, pain may be elicited with passive range of motion of the hip through flexion, adduction, and internal rotation. Pivoting on the affected leg may be painful or feel unstable. It is important to rule out iliopsoas syndrome as an etiology as this may also be positive for the above test.

Imaging/Diagnostic Evaluation   Standard radiographs can demonstrate associated acetabular dysplasia or degenerative changes of the hip, e.g. pincer and/or CAM impingement. Anterior posterior views of the pelvis and a true lateral of the hip should be obtained. MRI can reveal tears in the labrum similar to meniscal tears in the knee. MRA with 10–15 ml diluted gadolinium injected into the hip prior to imaging to detect labral tears is significantly more sensitive. Labral tears are still frequently missed on imaging, providing intra-articular lidocaine/corticosteroid injections and arthroscopy as reasonable diagnostic and therapeutic options.

Treatment   The treatment algorithm varies depending on the specific labral pathology. For an isolated labral tear, the dancer is initially instructed to limit dance activity that aggravates the pain and increases the stress placed on the hip joint for 4–6 weeks. For ballet dancers, this restriction includes limiting extreme hip external rotation. Restricted activity should be followed by an individualized physical therapy program once the pain symptoms resolve. Physical therapy should focus on iliopsoas and hip rotator stretching, strengthening, core stabilization and proprioception and balance training. The dancer should be carefully assessed for muscular imbalances and tightness. If the above options fail, consider a fluoroscopic guided intra-articular corticosteroid injection and/or oral anti-inflammatory medication as needed. Labral tears without pincer or CAM impingement usually do very well with arthroscopic debridement. Partial weight bearing may be instituted immediately post-operatively with full weight bearing usually occurring by 3–5 days post-operatively.

For a labral tear secondary to impingement, the patient should be evaluated by an orthopedic surgeon for labral repair via arthroscopic osteochondroplasty or debridement. Above average outcomes have been reported for patients without associated osteoarthritis or dysplasia, and outcomes in dancers have ranged from no relief to return to dance at their pre-operative level with an average of 6–8 months of rehabilitation. It has been suggested that similar to meniscal injuries in the knee, labral injuries with associated instability, subluxation, and excess joint loading can lead to arthritic joint changes.

References

1. Kellgren J, Lawrence J. Radiologic assessment of osteoarthritis. Ann Rheum Dis 1957; 16: 494–501.
2. Zhang W, Moskowitz RW, Nuki G et al. OARSI recommendations for the management of hip and knee osteoarthritis, Part II:OARSI evidence-based, expert consensus guidelines. Osteoarthr Cartilage 2008; 16(2): 137–62.
3. Robinson P, Keenan AM, Conaghan PG. Clinical effectiveness and dose response of image-guided intra-articular corticosteroid injection for hip osteoarthritis. Rheumatology 2007; 46: 285–91.
4. Micheli LJ. Dance injuries: The back, hip and pelvis. In PM Clarkson andM Skrinar (eds) Science of dance training 1988; 193–207. Champaign, IL. Human Kinetics..
5. Padgett DE. The unstable total hip replacement. Clin Ortho Rel Res 2004; 420: 72–79.
6. Adler RS, Buly R, Ambrose R, Sculco T. Diagnostic and therapeutic use of sonography-guided iliopsoas peritendinous injections. Am J Roentgenology 2005; 185: 940–43.
7. Rose DJ, Montalbano G, Rosen J et al. Iliopsoas syndrome in dancers. Med Sci Sports Exer 1998; 30(5)S: 288.
8. Schwarzer AC, Aprill CN, Bogduk N. The sacroiliac joint in chronic low back pain. Spine 1995; 20:31–37.
9. DeMann LE Jr. Sacroiliac dysfunction in dancers with low back pain. Manual Therapy 1997; 2(1): 2–10.
10. Cibulka MT, Sinacore DR, Cromer GS, Delitto A. Unilateral hip rotation range of motion asymmetry in patients with sacroiliac joint regional pain. Spine 1998; 23(9): 1009–15.
11. Dreyfuss P, Michaelsen M, Pauza K et al. The value of medical history and physical examination in diagnosing sacroiliac joint pain. Spine 1996; 21(22): 2594–602.
12. Mizuguchi T. Division of the piriformis muscle for the treatment of sciatica. Postlaminectomy syndrome and osteoarthritis of the spine. Arch Surg 1976; 111(6): 719–22.

5
Spine Injuries

Case Report   A 40-year-old modern dancer who was a gymnast in her teenage years presents to your office complaining of intermittent lower back pain for the past 6 months. It is worse with extension and bridges and does not radiate into the lower extremities.

Diagnosis   Lumbar zygapophysial joint (z-joint or facet) arthropathy

Epidemiology   Second most common source of low back pain.

Pathophysiology   Similar to most overuse injuries seen in dance, zygapophysial joint arthropathy usually develops over time as a result of the significant stress placed on the lumbar spine following repetitive hyperextension. Positions that increase lumbar extension, including *arabesque*, *attitude derrière* (Figures 5-1) in ballet and modern dance, bridges, back walk-overs, and back handsprings (Figures 5-2) in gymnastics exacerbate this condition. Z-joint arthropathy tends to develop in older dancers or those with many years of experience as a result of degenerative changes to the z-joints. Similar to osteoarthritis, the symptoms of degenerative z-joint disease include erosion of cartilage and the z-joint surfaces, narrowing of the z-joint space and development of osteophytes (also known as bone spurs) and/or subchondral sclerosis along the z-joint surfaces. In addition to the degenerative changes, one or more of the osteophytes or the z-joint itself may fracture during periods of increased dance activity.

History   The patient typically presents complaining of back pain worse with extension and turning to one side. The pain may be localized to the lower back or may radiate down the lower extremity if there is associated irritation of the nerve root adjacent to the z-joint. A referral pain pattern is typically dull, aching, and difficult to localize. Pain is usually insidious and may be worse with standing, descending stairs, and walking.

From: *Musculoskeletal Medicine*: *Essential Dance Medicine*
By A. Bracilović, DOI 10.1007/978-1-59745-546-6_5,
© Humana Press, a part of Springer Science+Business Media, LLC 2009

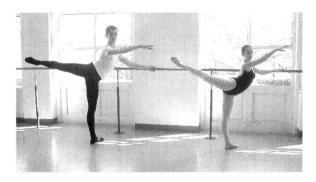

FIGURE 5-1. **(A)** *Arabesque*, flat.

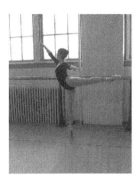

FIGURE 5-1. **(B)** *Arabesque*, on pointe.

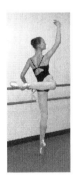

FIGURE 5-1. **(C)** *Attitude derrière*, on pointe.

PE   The patient may have tenderness to palpation over the lumbar z-joints and the surrounding paraspinal muscles on the affected side. Lumbar hyperextension with lateral rotation (oblique extension) to the involved side typically reproduces the pain. Dancers tend to utilize extreme ranges of motion of the lumbar spine; therefore, apparently "normal" range of motion on examination may be significantly decreased range of motion for a dancer (Figures 5-3 and 5-4).

The dancer's technique in lumbar extension is important to assess as patients will often incorrectly demonstrate lumbar hyperlordosis and lack

FIGURE 5-2. **(A)** Bridge.

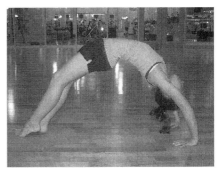

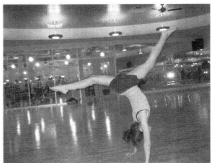

FIGURE 5-2. **(B)** Back walkover.

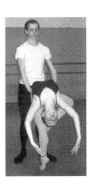

FIGURE 5-3. Spine range of motion.

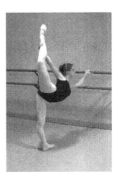

FIGURE 5-4. Spine, hip range of motion.

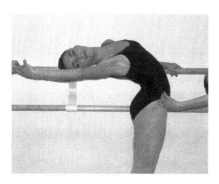

FIGURE 5-5. Exaggerated spine hyperextension.

of use of abdominal muscles in positions *en derrière* that increase lumbar extension. When at the barre and in center, the patient should be evaluated for proper positioning throughout full range of motion of the demonstrated exercise (Figure 5-5).

Imaging/Diagnostic Evaluation   Radiographs of the lumbar spine may show degenerative z-joint changes, including osteophytes, irregularity of the joint line, joint space narrowing, and/or subchondral sclerosis. CT and/ or MRI can demonstrate more specific degenerative changes of the z-joint but with questionable reliability. Bone scan with SPECT imaging has recently been used with increasing frequency to diagnose z-joint pathology. The gold standard with which to diagnose z-joint disease are fluoroscopic guided medial branch blocks. In double blind blocks, a short acting anesthetic such as lidocaine is first injected into the joint, followed by injection with a longer acting anesthetic such as bupivacaine.

Treatment   A carefully prescribed physical therapy regimen involving anti-lordotic exercises, core strengthening, and lumbar stabilization is essential for the acute as well as maintenance phase, and to prevent recurrence of symptoms. Should physical therapy fail, consider an intra-articular injection of corticosteroid and anesthetic. Relief from this injection can be diagnostic as well as therapeutic. If the patient experiences no relief from the injection and the specific z-joint or joints have been identified as the pain generators, radiofrequency neurotomy of the medial branches of the dorsal rami innervating the involved z-joints may be performed under fluoroscopic guidance. Surgical excision of any fractured osteophytes, if present, or excision of the z-joint itself is considered only if the above treatment options fail. Spinal fusion is considered only as a last resort.

Case Report   A 30-year-old male ballet dancer presents to your office complaining of pain in his lower back when bending forward while sitting and when lifting most objects heavier than a few pounds. He initially felt the pain during a performance, then again after practicing a lift with a fellow company member.

Diagnosis   Discogenic pain

Epidemiology   More common in male than female dancers secondary to increased pressure on discs during lifts.

Pathophysiology   Low back pain can arise from injury to the lumbar intervertebral discs. The outer third of the annulus fibrosus of lumbar discs is richly innervated and when a radial tear or fissure extends into the outer third of the annulus, nociceptive nerve endings in the annulus fibrosus can be stimulated chemically as well as mechanically, resulting in the clinical symptom of low back pain. Internal disc disruption refers to disruption of the disc without external bulge or herniation. If an annular tear extends into the periphery of the annulus fibrosus in the vicinity of a degraded nucleus pulposus, the nucleus can herniate if the disc is under compression. A visual analogy is squeezing jelly (nucleus pulposus) out of a donut (annulus fibrosus).

In dancers, mechanical compression of the disc increases with frequent forward lumbar flexion, which significantly increases the load placed on lumbar discs when compared to the load in neutral position. Also, in male dancers, this load on the discs is further increased when carrying the weight of another dancer in the arms or when the flexed spine is rotated. This load is increased when the arms are held away from the body (Figure 5-6). Poor technique with lumbar hyperlordosis is also frequently associated with inadequate lifting strength and core instability (Figures 5-7).

If the extruded nucleus herniates centrally, pain can be felt in the lower back. If the nucleus herniates laterally, it can irritate nerve roots that supply the leg. Irritation of the nerve roots can also cause numbness or tingling in

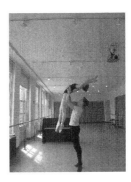

FIGURE 5-6. Increased lumbar load with hands held away from body.

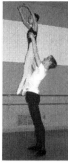

FIGURE 5-7. **(A)** Hyperlordosis.

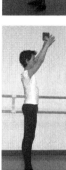

FIGURE 5-7. **(B)** Improved hyperlordosis.

the leg or muscle weakness. These signs of neurologic loss are reflective of a radiculopathy, which will be discussed in the next section.

History   The patient will typically complain of low back pain, worse with bending forward, sitting, or lifting from a seated or standing position. He or she may report an acute incident, often involving lifting or lifting and twisting using incorrect technique. It may be exacerbated with coughing, sneezing, or any activity that increases intradiscal pressure. If there is an associated radiculopathy, the patient may report symptoms of motor weakness or numbness and/or tingling in the lower extremities.

PE   Although no physical exam finding is pathognomonic for discogenic low back pain, a thorough musculoskeletal and neurologic physical examination is important to further corroborate the information obtained from the patient's history and symptoms. Depending on the acuity of the pain, the patient may have tenderness to palpation of the lumbar paraspinal muscles that are in spasm, decreased active range of motion in lumbar flexion secondary to pain and tight hamstrings and/or hip flexors. Without associated pain generators in addition to the disc, the neurologic examination should be intact.

Imaging/Diagnostic Evaluation   While MRI is the best non-invasive imaging technique to visualize degenerative changes within the disc, including tears in the annulus, the correlation between changes seen on MRI and the existence of patient's symptoms is not direct. In other words, a patient having low back pain symptoms may or may not have identifiable disc pathology to explain the source of their pain, and patients with demonstrable disc pathology on MRI may not have pain corresponding to their MRI findings. The gold standard for diagnosing internal disc disruption is disc stimulation and post-discography CT. Stimulation of the disc identifies which disc is painful and post-discography CT delineates the morphology of the nucleus and presence of an annular tear.

Treatment   In young dancers, the natural history of disc herniations tends to be resorption of the herniated disc over the course of weeks to months. For acute pain, a course of anti-inflammatory medications or muscle relaxants is initially used. An individualized physical therapy program should focus first on correcting improper alignment and biomechanics, improving segmental motion and progress to an anti-lordotic stretching, strengthening and core stabilization program. Education regarding proper activation of the abdominal and lumbar paraspinal musculature and correct pelvic alignment during lifts, at the barre and in center is essential for core strengthening and prevention of injury. A brace or corset together with the exercise program can help immobilize the lumbar spine. Surgical excision is considered only as a last resort if the patient's symptoms are not responsive to non-operative treatment.

Case Report   A 27-year-old modern dancer performing in the Broadway production of "STOMP" presents to your office complaining of low back pain associated with radiating pain down the back of his leg and occasionally into the side of his foot.

Diagnosis   Lumbar radiculopathy and radicular pain

Epidemiology   L5 most common radiculopathy in lumbar spine.

Pathophysiology   A radiculopathy is defined as a state of neurologic loss in which conduction is blocked in the axons of a spinal nerve or its roots. In sensory axons, this conduction block results in numbness and in motor axons, weakness. These symptoms occur as a result of compression or ischemia of axons of a spinal nerve root. They reflect an inflammatory process that involves nerve root swelling and toxic injury. The most common causes of a radiculopathy include a herniated disc (most common), foraminal stenosis, epidural disorders such as infection or lipoma, meningeal disorders, and neurologic disorders, including but not limited to diabetes, cysts, infection, and tumors.

In distinguishing between a radiculopathy, radicular pain, and referred pain, it is important to remember that a radiculopathy reflects a state of neurologic loss that may or may not be associated with radicular pain. Radicular pain refers to a shooting, electric, radiating pain that occurs secondary to compression of a dorsal root ganglion or mechanical compression combined with chemical irritation and inflammation of a spinal nerve root. The two entities can occur together or separately. Referred pain is often described as dull, deep, aching, and difficult to localize. It arises as a result of the brain misattributing the source of pain from separate distal sites whose neural pathways converge in the same area of the brain. The pain is perceived in a region other than the pathologic source of pain. Symptoms that sound like referred pain may be radicular, but symptoms that are radicular are not referred. These are important to distinguish, as management differs for both.

In the lumbar spine, an L5 radiculopathy is common and may occur most often secondary to the tight fit of the root in its foramen. The L5 nerve root has the largest diameter and narrowest intervertebral foramen.

History   In the lumbar spine, the patient may complain of low back pain with associated leg pain, numbness, tingling, or weakness. Depending on the nerve root involved, the symptoms may involve the anterior, posterior, lateral, or medial aspects of the thigh, lower leg, and/or foot.

It is also important when evaluating the patient for a radiculopathy to assess for any red flag symptoms. These include fever, weight loss, chills, and any history of tumor. Adolescent patients and those greater than 50 years old are at increased risk for back pain of a malignant etiology, including tumor and infection. In the cervical and thoracic spine, intraspinal tumors can compress the spinal cord as well as the nerve roots and present as a myeloradiculopathy. It is important to remember that compression of the spinal cord is a medical emergency and to always ask about recent bowel or bladder dysfunction, significant lower extremity deficits in strength or sensation and the presence of saddle anesthesia. Any of these symptoms require urgent medical attention.

PE   The patient should have a thorough musculoskeletal and neurologic examination, including evaluation of motor strength, sensation, and reflexes. Active range of motion of the lumbar spine may be reduced secondary to pain. Tenderness to palpation or muscle spasm may be noted along the lumbar paraspinals. Assess for upper motor neuron signs, including spasticity, clonus, Babinski reflex, and Hoffman's sign.

The straight leg raise can be performed with the patient lying supine and passively flexing the uninvolved hip. Passively extend the symptomatic leg. At 35–70 degrees of extended leg elevation, the nerves are maximally stretched and can reproduce the patient's symptoms (Figure 5-8). The sitting slump or dural tension test is performed with the patient in a seated position with the head, upper chest, and shoulders in a forward slumped position, to increase the stretch on the sciatic nerve (Figure 5-9). This test evaluates L5-S1 radicular symptoms and is considered positive when symptoms radiating down the leg are reproduced, *not* with hamstring tightness.

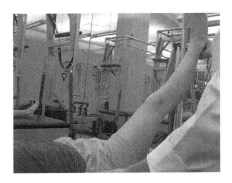

FIGURE 5-8. Straight leg raise.

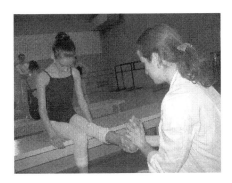

FIGURE 5-9. Dural tension test.

Imaging/Diagnostic Evaluation For herniations in the lumbar spine, radiographs are usually unremarkable and are more useful to detect structural pathology. MRI is indicated to specify the level of pathology and in patients whose symptoms are not responding to therapy, who have progressive neurologic deficits or evidence of cauda equina syndrome. CT and myelogram are typically indicated for pre-operative patients, those with progressive neurologic deficits and when MRI and electromyogram (EMG) are not diagnostic. Nerve conduction studies and needle EMG are useful to diagnose nerve root dysfunction when the diagnosis is uncertain or to distinguish radiculopathy from other lesions, such as peripheral neuropathy or plexopathy. In the second week post-injury, positive sharp waves and fibrillations can first be seen in proximal, followed by distal, muscles. Therefore, the study should be delayed until 3 weeks but less than 6 months following injury to increase the likelihood of obtaining informative results.

Treatment The natural history of radiculopathy secondary to disc herniations is eventual resorption of the disc and improvement in the patient's symptoms. Treatment initially consists of an individualized physical therapy program focused on lumbar stabilization and core strengthening. Manipulation, soft tissue mobilization, and lumbar traction to distract the vertebral bodies have also been used. Perhaps the most essential component of the physical therapy program to prevent further injury is institution and adherence to a home exercise program, which the patient can incorporate into their regular schedule. NSAIDs are useful to treat pain and inflammation, while muscle relaxants can be used for radiculopathy associated with muscles in acute spasm. Opioids and anticonvulsants such as gabapentin and pregabalin are approved for neuropathic pain.

For pain that does not resolve with physical therapy and medications, consider an epidural steroid injection for a carefully identified population of patients. These injections can be administered via transforaminal, interlaminar, and caudal routes. Surgery is indicated for significant and progressive motor deficits, or cauda equina syndrome with bowel and bladder dysfunction. Surgical options include percutaneous discectomy, microdiscectomy, discectomy with or without fusion, chemonucleolysis, laminectomy, or laminotomy for patients with spinal stenosis.

Case Report   A 14-year-old female ballet student presents to your office complaining of delayed menarche and a "rib hump" noted by her mother. She denies associated back pain or other medical problems.

Diagnosis   Scoliosis

Epidemiology   Higher prevalence in dancers than in the general population.

Pathophysiology   Scoliosis involves a three dimensional deformity of the spinal segments with lateral curvature and vertebral body rotation. It can occur in any segment of the spine and has been divided into different categories depending on the age of onset: congenital, infantile, juvenile, adolescent, and adult. It can also be described as occurring secondary to a preexisting condition, such as cerebral palsy. Most often the cause of scoliosis is idiopathic; however, a gene has been recently identified in association with idiopathic scoliosis [1]. Congenital scoliosis may result from abnormal development of the spine during embryonic development and may be associated with neurologic deficits. Infantile scoliosis is described in patients less than 3 years old and is typically associated with congenital defects. Juvenile scoliosis is described in patients 4–10 years old and is often associated with a high risk of curve progression. In dancers, adolescent idiopathic is the most common type and is characterized for patients 11 years old to growth completion. It is also associated with a high risk of curve progression, occurs with equal frequency in males and females, although the risk of curve progression is greater in females. During the adolescent growth spurt, the rate of curve progression is approximately 1 degree per month.

History   Scoliosis in and of itself is not a direct cause of back pain and the patient will not typically complain of back pain secondary to scoliosis. In ballet dancers, delayed menarche and prolonged episodes of amenorrhea have been suggested as predisposing factors for scoliosis; therefore, it is very important to elicit a patient's menstrual history.

PE   On physical examination, first assess the patient's gait and check the feet for cavovarus deformity. It is also important to evaluate for asymmetry at various levels. Inspect the patient for shoulder height asymmetry, a prominent scapula, protruding ribs, and asymmetric iliac crest heights. Evaluate the patient's range of motion in lumbar flexion, extension, and lateral rotation. The Adam's bending test is used to assess appropriate rotation of the ribcage in thoracic scoliosis. If the patient has visible asymmetry of the ribs in forward lumbar flexion seen as an asymmetric prominence of the posterior trunk, the test is positive and scoliosis should be suspected (Figure 5-10). Thoracic curvature to the right, or dextroscoliosis, is most common and can usually be visualized at the T7 or T8 level. Levoscoliosis describes curvature to the left.

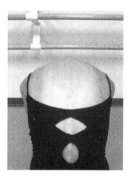

FIGURE 5-10. Adam's bending test.

Imaging/Diagnostic Evaluation   AP, lateral, and scoliosis views obtained posteriorly can reveal scoliotic curvature. Typically, the Cobb angle is the standard measurement used to quantitatively determine the degree of spine curvature. The Cobb angle refers to the angle between two intersecting perpendicular lines drawn from the superior border of the first endplate noted to have curvature and the inferior border of the most inferiorly involved endplate. If multiple curves are noted, Cobb angles are drawn for each curve. The degree of vertebral body rotation is measured by evaluating the position of the pedicle and is graded from 0 (no rotation) to 4 (complete rotation where the contralateral pedicle is shifted past midline). Serial radiographs are typically obtained in patients who are still growing to follow curve progression, approximately every 3–6 months.

Treatment   Treatment of scoliosis typically falls into one of three possible options: observation, orthosis, or operative management. The choice of treatment option depends on the severity of the curve. If the curve is less than 20 degrees, treatment typically begins with observation of curve progression and an individualized physical therapy program that focuses on flexibility exercises, joint mobilization, and stretching and strengthening exercises to lengthen shortened muscles and strengthen overemphasized muscles. Emphasis is also given to proper posture and biomechanical alignment in dance as well as everyday activities.

Orthosis options are recommended when the curve is between 20 and 40 degrees and typically include a custom-molded cervical-thoracic-lumbar-sacral orthosis (CTLSO) or thoraco-lumbosacral orthosis (TLSO). Orthoses are worn 23 hours per day until the end of the patient's growth spurt. The Milwaukee brace is a type of CTLSO and the Boston brace is a type of TLSO. The effectiveness of bracing is highly dependent upon patient compliance, and it is important to remind patients to wear the brace as often as possible, including during dance activities. In young children, orthoses may prevent progression of severe curves and can potentially delay surgery on the spine of a growing child. If the degree of curvature is greater than 40 degrees in a growing patient, surgical correction is indicated, most often with spinal fusion.

Case Report   A 16-year-old female gymnast and ballet dancer presents to your office complaining of low back pain that began gradually and is worse with arabesque, attitude, back walk-overs, and back handsprings.

Diagnosis   Spondylolysis

Epidemiology   Greater incidence in gymnasts and female Caucasian dancers [2]. Thought to have hereditary predisposition.

Pathophysiology   Spondylolysis typically arises as one of several spinal overuse injuries seen in dancers. It represents a defect in the normal bony structure of the pars interarticularis, most commonly in the lumbar spine at the L5 level. It typically occurs as a result of microtrauma from repetitive hyperextension and rotation of the lumbar spine. If the fracture occurs bilaterally, the superior vertebra may slip over the inferior vertebra, causing spondylolisthesis (see below).

In ballet dancers, frequent hyperextension of the lumbar spine in arabesque, attitude, and other movements involving leg extension greater than 90 degrees can stress any of the posterior elements of the lumbar spine and specifically shear the pars, causing a stress fracture to occur. Often, ballet dancers who attempt to compensate for less than ideal turnout from their hips will instead go into hyperlordosis with increased anterior pelvic tilt. This removes some tension from the anterior hip capsule ligaments, especially the iliofemoral ligament, after which the dancer will typically force turnout from their feet and attempt to increase external rotation at their hips [3].

History   The dancer may present with low back pain that started gradually and is localized to the affected side (if unilateral). The pain is typically worse with *arabesque*, *attitude*, and *grand battement derrière* (Figures 5-11). Pain is also noticed when standing on the affected side with the lumbar spine hyperextended. Usually, the patient does not report associated numbness, tingling, weakness, or radiating pain down the lower extremity.

FIGURE 5-11. **(A)** Arabesque, flat.

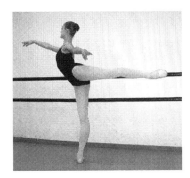

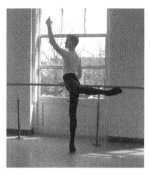

FIGURE 5-11. **(B)** Attitude derrière.

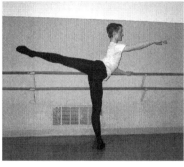

FIGURE 5-11. **(C)** Grand battement derrière.

PE   On exam, the patient may have full range of motion in lumbar flexion, extension and lateral rotation or slightly limited lumbar flexion if the hamstrings are tight. Dancers typically have above average flexibility, so decreased range of motion may not be elicited. Hyperextension of the spine is typically painful, in arabesque, attitude, and especially when the patient stands on the affected side. **Pain elicited with extension is spondylolysis in a dancer or gymnast until proven otherwise.** The surrounding paraspinal muscles may be in spasm. The patient may be able to localize a specific area of pain.

Imaging/Diagnostic Evaluation   While AP radiographs are typically normal, oblique views can demonstrate a defect in the pars that may resemble a stress fracture. The pars defect will appear as a break in the neck or the collar of the "Scotty dog." Single photon emission computerized tomography (SPECT) bone scan can demonstrate increased activity at the involved regions and is useful for identifying acute stress reactions prior to their appearance on radiographs. CT will demonstrate detailed evidence of fractures and other bony pathology.

Treatment   In the acute phase, immobilization of the symptomatic area with bracing and physical therapy are recommended until the injury heals or the patient no longer has symptoms with dance activity. The brace is typically worn in neutral lordosis (0 degrees) for 23 hours daily until the patient is free of symptoms. A bone scan is usually repeated after a minimum of 3 months.

Physical therapy should focus on hamstring, iliopsoas, paraspinal, and abdominal muscle stretching, which can be done while in the brace. Hyperextension should be avoided. Although the fracture may not heal completely by radiographic evaluation, the dancer can be allowed to return to dance after the symptoms resolve. Fibrous healing of the fracture can coincide with complete resolution of the patient's symptoms.

Case Report   A 14-year-old female gymnast and modern dancer presents to your office complaining of lower back pain while doing backbends, back walk-overs, and back handsprings during gymnastics practice and while doing bridges in modern dance class rehearsal. She describes the pain as dull and aching, occasionally extending to her buttocks. It is improved with sitting.

Diagnosis   Spondylolisthesis

Epidemiology   Occurs most often at the L4–L5 level.

Pathophysiology   Spondylolisthesis describes anterior translation of one superior vertebral body upon the vertebral body immediately inferior to it. Depending on the cause of the spondylolisthesis, the type of translation is described differently. Five categories have been described. The first category (Type I) refers to congenital spondylolisthesis, which is characterized by anterior translation of dysplastic sacral zygapophysial joints. Type II describes a stress fracture of the pars interarticularis causing isthmic spondylolisthesis, which is typically seen in dancers and gymnasts. Type III describes degenerative spondylolisthesis that arises from zygapophysial joint disease that causes intersegmental instability. Acute trauma to the pars interarticularis causes type IV spondylolisthesis. Pathologic spondylolisthesis arises from any destabilizing injury to the zygapophysial joints.

Spondylolisthesis is also graded according to the percentage of anterior displacement of the superior vertebral body to the superior end plate of the inferior vertebral body. Grade 1 describes 1–25% displacement, grade 2 26–50%, grade 3 51–75%, grade 4 76–100%, and grade 5 greater than 100% displacement.

History   Depending on the cause of spondylolisthesis, the history of a patient's symptoms may differ. The presentation is almost identical to spondylolysis. Type II spondylolisthesis occurs more often in dancers than other types. The patient may complain of mild pain initially with dance activity, particularly in lumbar extension, such as *arabesque*, *attitude*, and *grand battement derrière*; however, often the patient does not have preceding pain symptoms. If the patient has pain, it may be acute or gradual in nature. Traumatic spondylolisthesis is associated with acute trauma, pain and may result in spinal cord compression. Other types of spondylolisthesis do not typically cause neurologic symptoms.

PE   The physical examination findings may be similar to that of spondylolysis. The patient who presents with isthmic spondylolisthesis may have a palpable lumbar step-off if the spondylolisthesis is grade 2 or greater. The lumbar paraspinals may also be tender to palpation and in spasm. Often, dancers will have loss of hamstring flexibility.

Imaging/Diagnostic Evaluation   AP, standing lateral, oblique, and flexion/extension radiographs are useful to demonstrate the degree of displacement. SPECT is helpful to distinguish a hot from a cold lesion. Otherwise, a lesion that is no longer metabolically active does not require bracing. CT can demonstrate any associated bony pathology and CT with myelogram and MRI will demonstrate the presence of nerve root compression and central or foraminal stenosis.

Treatment   Depending on the grade of spondylolisthesis, management differs. For dancers with an acute isthmic lesion, dance activity should be restricted until the patient is symptom free. An individualized physical therapy program should focus on improving hamstring flexibility and abdominal strength. Exercises to decrease lumbar hyperlordosis, avoid lumbar hyperextension, and increase core stability are essential. A fracture that is healing will be positive on bone scan and can be treated with bracing. Serial radiographs should be performed for patients with isthmic or congenital spondylolisthesis approximately every 6 months. Rarely does displacement progress following adolescence.

Patients with degenerative spondylolisthesis are also typically treated conservatively and present as older patients who may require treatment for additional medical problems. Pathologic spondylolisthesis management should include appropriate diagnostic work-up to direct treatment. Traumatic spondylolisthesis often require surgical intervention when the patient presents with neurologic symptoms and/or back pain symptoms that do not resolve with conservative management. Spondylolisthesis greater than 50% (grade 3 and above) and traumatic spondylolisthesis typically require surgical intervention.

Case Report A 24-year-old male ballet dancer presents to your office complaining of lower back pain that began gradually and is worse when lifting his partner overhead. He had been instructed to start weight training for "core strengthening" although he admits he has little time to spend in the gym and finds weightlifting boring.

Diagnosis   Mechanical low back pain

Epidemiology More common in dancers with hyperlordotic posture and lack of core strength.

Pathophysiology Low back pain that is described as mechanical refers generally to etiologies that are somatic in origin, resulting from stimulation of nociceptive nerve endings in bone, joints, ligaments, muscles of the lumbar spine or some combination thereof. These etiologies typically exclude visceral causes in which the source of pain is a body organ or neurogenic causes in which the pain arises from pathology of peripheral nerve cell bodies or axons. Non-mechanical causes can also be systemic, such as infection, osteoporosis, and metastatic disease. It is usually a diagnosis of exclusion, once more specific causes have been ruled out.

In dancers, mechanical low back pain typically arises from a combination of poor posture, hyperlordosis, weakness of abdominal muscles, and tight hamstrings and lumbar fascia. There may be associated ligamentous sprain or muscular strain, usually secondary to poor posture and biomechanical alignment. Ballet dancers are particularly at risk for mechanical low back pain secondary to the increased tendency to attempt to improve external rotation from the hips. The dancer will anteriorly tilt the pelvis to slacken the anterior hip ligaments, force turnout from the feet upward, and hyperextend the lumbar spine. This places excessive strain on the posterior lumbar extensor muscles and underutilizes the abdominal and pelvic floor muscles, which are usually weak. Hyperlordosis occurs as a result with subsequent compression of the vertebrae and hypercontraction of the surrounding extensor muscles.

Adolescent dancers may also experience their growth spurts "asymmetrically," where the vertebral bony components of the spine develop faster than the surrounding tendons and ligaments, resulting in tightness of the hamstrings and lumbar fascia. This exacerbates the hyperlordosis that may already exist from poor technique.

History The young dancer typically presents as an adolescent, with low back pain that is worse with dance activity. The pain may be localized and exacerbated by specific movements, or may be more diffuse, aching, and difficult to pinpoint. It is usually worse with lumbar hyperextension and associated with poor posture and technique.

PE Physical examination may reproduce pain in lumbar hyperextension or in multiple directions with active range of motion. The musculoskeletal and neurologic examinations are usually normal and any associated provocative maneuvers for more specific etiologies, i.e. sitting slump or dural tension test, straight leg raise, sacroiliac joint tenderness, referred pain patterns, etc., should be negative. There may be associated hamstring tightness and weak abdominal muscles.

Imaging/Diagnostic Evaluation   Diagnostic and imaging studies should be ordered if other specific etiologies are suspected. Disc herniations, infection, tumors, etc. should be excluded with appropriate evaluation prior to making the diagnosis of mechanical low back pain.

Treatment   It is important to establish proper posture, alignment, and correct dance technique at the barre, center and for lifting, if applicable. An individualized physical therapy program should focus on reducing hyperlordosis, strengthening abdominal and pelvic floor muscles, stretching the hamstrings and posterior lumbar extensor muscles, and correctly utilizing the dancer's degree of turnout, or external rotation at the hips. If specific exercises do not alleviate the pain and correct the patient's biomechanics over time, an anti-lordotic brace may be considered to supplement the therapy program. The brace is normally worn at all times except during dance activity for approximately 6–12 weeks, then gradually decreased in duration for 3–4 months until the patient can dance without pain. Emphasis should be placed on maintaining appropriate biomechanical alignment, correct lifting technique (especially for male dancers), and avoiding hyperlordosis long term even after the patient is free of symptoms.

Case Report   A 29-year-old male ballet dancer presents to your office complaining of neck and arm pain radiating down into his hand, mainly into the middle finger. He initially felt the pain during a performance while lifting his partner overhead. He occasionally has pain in the lateral aspect of his shoulder and believes some of his hand feels numb at times.

Diagnosis   Cervical radiculopathy and radicular pain

Epidemiology   C7 most common radiculopathy in cervical spine.

Pathophysiology   Please refer to the Pathophysiology section of lumbar radiculopathy.

History   In evaluating a patient for a cervical radiculopathy, it is important to distinguish the neurologic causes of pain from non-neurologic etiologies. In the cervical spine, the patient may complain of insidious onset of neck and arm discomfort associated with radiating, shooting, electric pain down the arm in a band-like pattern. There may be associated sensory changes along the involved nerve root sclerotome, such as tingling, numbness, or loss of sensation. Motor weakness in the upper extremity may also be present.

It is also important when evaluating the patient for a radiculopathy to assess for any red flag symptoms. These include fever, weight loss, chills, and any history of tumor. Adolescent patients and those greater than 50 years old are at increased risk for back pain of a malignant etiology, including tumor and infection. In the cervical and thoracic spine, intraspinal tumors can compress the spinal cord as well as the nerve roots and present as a myeloradiculopathy. It is important to remember that compression of the spinal cord is a medical emergency and to always ask about recent bowel or bladder dysfunction, significant lower extremity deficits in strength or sensation and the presence of saddle anesthesia. All of these symptoms require urgent medical attention.

PE   The patient should have a thorough musculoskeletal and neurologic examination, including evaluation of motor strength, sensation, and reflexes. Active range of motion of the cervical spine may be reduced. Tenderness to palpation or muscle spasm may be noted along the cervical paraspinals. Assess for upper motor neuron signs, including spasticity, Babinski, and Hoffman's sign. In the cervical spine, perform Spurling's test to evaluate foraminal compression [4]. This provocative maneuver is performed by extending the neck and rotating the head to the suspected side of the pathology and applying axial compression. The maneuver is considered positive when radicular symptoms are reproduced down the arm. Patients with cervical radiculopathy will also typically have pain relief with abduction of the ipsilateral shoulder and placing the hand on the head (shoulder abduction sign). Sensation and/or reflexes in the upper extremity may be diminished. Motor weakness may be a result of significant root compromise or may be secondary to pain. In dancers, it is also

FIGURE 5-12. **(A)** Cervical kyphosis.

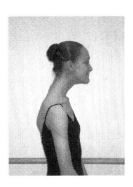

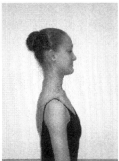

FIGURE 5-12. **(B)** Cervical kyphosis corrected.

important to assess posture and positioning of the neck and upper back as well as scapulohumeral alignment and range of motion (Figures 5-12). Proper scapular kinematics, cervical spine posture, and adequate proprioception are essential to prevent injury.

Imaging/Diagnostic Evaluation For the cervical spine, standard radiographs are useful to detect degenerative changes, fractures, subluxation, and gross bony pathology. Any history of trauma should include AP, lateral, bilateral oblique, flexion, extension, and open-mouth views. CT with myelography will demonstrate the integrity of the spinal canal and can reveal spinal cord compression. MRI is the method of choice to localize nerve root impingement and to assess the integrity of the disc, vertebral bodies, and surrounding soft tissue. Nerve conduction studies and EMG are helpful to differentiate cervical radiculopathy from other neuropathic conditions such as plexopathy, peripheral neuropathy, or carpal tunnel syndrome.

Treatment The natural history of cervical radiculopathy is unclear. Initially, relative rest from dance activity for 3–5 days and NSAIDs are recommended to reduce pain, inflammation, and specifically nerve root irritation and edema. Some advise use of a soft cervical collar or cervical pillow at night to help prevent neck movement and maintain a neutral position. Manual and self-powered traction can be used, although it is important to avoid neck extension.

In the acute phase, therapy should include isometric exercises to strengthen the muscles affected by the radiculopathy. Low weight with more frequent repetitions as well as closed kinetic chain exercises are recommended for weak shoulder girdle muscles. After the pain and inflammation are controlled, physical therapy should be advanced to restore full range of motion. Exercises should then progress to isotonic strengthening once the radicular symptoms are improved. For cervical radiculopathies, scapular stabilization exercises and manual resistive cervical stabilization exercises in various planes are important. Soft tissue mobilization techniques are useful to stretch the non-contractile elements. NSAIDs are helpful to reduce pain and inflammation. Tricyclic antidepressants may be used as adjunct medications to control radicular pain. Opioids are typically not necessary or recommended unless other regimens fail or are contraindicated. When the above treatment options fail, consider cervical epidural steroid injections. Surgical options are recommended only as a last resort. It is recommended for cervical instability, for patients with symptoms of progressive neurologic deficits, long tract signs, and failure to improve following injections.

References

1. Warren MP, Brooks-Gunn J, Hamilton LH et al. Scoliosis and fractures in young ballet dancers. Relation to delayed menarche and secondary amenorrhea. New Eng J Med 1986; 314(21): 1348–53.
2. Jackson DW, Wiltse LL, Cirincione RJ. Spondylolysis in the female gymnast. Clin Orth 1976; 117: 68–73.
3. Solomon R, Brown T, Gerbino PG, Michel LJ. Pediatric and adolescent sports injuries: The young dancer. Clin Sports Med 2000; 19(4): 717–39.
4. Spurling RG. Lesions of the cervical intervertebral disc. Springfield, IL: Charles Thomas, 1956.

6
Shoulder Injuries

Case Report   A 36-year-old male modern dancer presents to your office complaining of pain over the top of his shoulder following a fall onto his arm and shoulder. The pain is worse when trying to wrap his scarf around his neck.

Diagnosis   Acromioclavicular (AC) joint sprain

Epidemiology   Typically occurs following a fall onto the shoulder or from direct force on the shoulder.

Pathophysiology   The acromioclavicular ligament attaches the distal end of the clavicle to the acromion and provides horizontal joint stability, as opposed to the coracoclavicular ligament, which provides vertical AC joint stability. A fall onto the arm and shoulder or direct injury to the shoulder is the usual mechanism of injury and can result in one of six types of AC joint injury. Type I involves a partial sprain of the AC ligament, no injury to the coracoclavicular (CC) ligament, and no clavicular displacement. A type II injury involves a complete AC ligament tear, partial CC tear, and no clavicular displacement. A type III injury involves complete AC and CC ligament tears and superior clavicular displacement. A type IV injury involves complete AC and CC ligament tears and posterosuperior clavicular displacement. A type V injury involves complete AC and CC ligament tears, posterosuperior clavicular displacement, deltoid and trapezius disruption and doubling of the coracoclavicular space. A type VI injury involves complete AC and CC ligament tears as well as inferior clavicular displacement.

History   The patient will typically complain of superior shoulder pain over the AC joint, worse with attempted adduction of the arm across midline. Any suspicion for AC joint separation should prompt referral to an orthopedic surgeon.

From: *Musculoskeletal Medicine*: *Essential Dance Medicine*
By A. Bracilović, DOI 10.1007/978-1-59745-546-6_6,
© Humana Press, a part of Springer Science+Business Media, LLC 2009

PE   Physical examination will typically reveal tenderness to palpation over the AC joint and decreased active and passive range of motion with the arm adducted past midline. The "scarf" test is considered positive when the patient has tenderness to palpation over the AC joint as the examiner passively adducts the patient's arm across midline.

Imaging/Diagnostic Evaluation   AP radiographs of the shoulder with the patient bearing weight (10 lbs) should be obtained. Type V injuries can show more than 100% expansion of the coracoclavicular region and type III injuries can show 25–100% widening.

Treatment   Management of acromioclavicular joint sprains depends on the degree of injury. Type I and II injuries typically require **PRICE** initially and the patient should avoid lifting of significant weight (including partners in dance) as well as any applied force to the affected shoulder. A type I injury typically requires about 2 weeks prior to return to dance activity and a type II injury may require up to 6 weeks off from dance. A sling may be worn for comfort for 2–4 weeks. The patient should be allowed to return to class and rehearsal when free of symptoms and full range of shoulder motion is regained.

Beginning with type III injuries, either non-operative or operative management may be considered, depending on the patient's dance or other occupational requirements. Cosmetics may play a part in this as well for a female dancer. Occasional gross cosmetic deformities may also be considered for surgical intervention, although dancers may trade a bump for an incisional scar.

Patients with type III injuries should be referred to an orthopedic surgeon for evaluation.

Usually, elite dancers who require high level function of the shoulder joint may require surgical management, especially for chronic instability or pain. For chronic AC joint pain or for patients who are not surgical candidates, an intra-articular corticosteroid injection may be helpful. Patients with associated AC joint arthritis may also benefit from an intra-articular lidocaine injection, combined with a focused physical therapy program. Patients should be allowed to return to dance activity when free of symptoms with manual traction with full range of shoulder motion and no tenderness to palpation at the AC joint. For types IV–VI, operative management is usually recommended, which typically includes open reduction internal fixation or distal resection of the clavicle with CC ligament reconstruction [1].

Case Report   A 30-year-old male ballet dancer presents to your office complaining of pain down the lateral aspect of his arm and in his shoulder, especially when lifting his partner or any object overhead.

Diagnosis   Shoulder impingement syndrome, rotator cuff tendonitis and tear

Epidemiology   Common cause of shoulder pain with repetitive overhead arm movements. Partial thickness tears common in young athletes can be asymptomatic in older adults.

Pathophysiology   Shoulder impingement occurs when the subacromial joint space is narrowed secondary to a number of possible inciting factors. The subacromial joint space is bordered by the coracoacromial arch and the rotator cuff. The coracoacromial arch is comprised of the coracoid process, the coracoacromial ligament and the acromion. The possible inciting factors may be anatomic or structural, acquired or congenital, including a congenitally curved or hooked acromion that narrows the joint space. Most often, repetitive microtrauma is the cause of impingement in dancers.

The rotator cuff is comprised of the supraspinatus, infraspinatus, teres minor, and subscapularis muscles. These four muscles hold the humeral head within the glenoid socket. The supraspinatus abducts the arm and depresses the humeral head. The infraspinatus and teres minor externally rotate and extend the arm, and the subscapularis internally rotates it. A rotator cuff tear can occur from acute trauma or as a result of some combination of external and internal factors including chronic repetitive microtrauma, subacromial impingement, and intrinsic tendon degeneration. The development of chronic microtrauma and subacromial impingement is thought to be affected by the shape of the acromion, with curved and hooked acromions associated with joint space narrowing and increased rotator cuff tear risk.

Dancers in particular maximally utilize the shoulder's wide range of motion, which can coincide with increased stress on its static and dynamic stabilizers, leading to instability and ultimately impingement. Repetitive overhead arm movements, as seen with male dancers lifting a partner, can irritate the underlying rotator cuff muscles with resultant inflammation, swelling, and compression of the subacromial bursa and rotator cuff muscles and tendons. The supraspinatus tendon is most frequently involved, as the area of impingement is localized over the supraspinatus tendon insertion on the superior facet of the greater tubercle of the humerus. High velocity eccentric extension movements also predispose for the development of impingement. Furthermore, if the dancer presents with weak rotator cuff muscles and shoulder instability, the shoulder joint will sustain a disproportionately larger stress than it can handle. If the muscles stabilizing the shoulder are not strong enough to hold the humeral head within its socket and are subject to overuse, the humeral head may move superiorly and impinge the subacromial space. If allowed to progress, subacromial impingement may lead to a partial or complete rotator cuff tear. Multiple partial tears can be associated with degenerative tendinopathy.

Subacromial impingement is typically divided into three stages. The first stage is most common in young dancers. It typically occurs in patients less than 25 years old, is reversible, and involves acute inflammation, edema, and hemorrhage of the rotator cuff and surrounding structures. The second stage involves tendonitis of the involved tendon(s) and may progress to fibrosis. It most commonly occurs in 25–40-year-old patients. The third stage involves a rotator cuff tear and is associated with acromioclavicular spurs. The third stage is most frequently seen in patients older than 40 years.

History   As dancers typically try to "work through" the pain, the patient will often come to the office well after the initial symptoms have started. The dancer complains of increased pain in the shoulder joint that may or may not extend into the lateral aspect of the arm and is worse with overhead activities. The pain is usually of gradual onset and associated with overuse, without a single inciting event. The pain may be associated with a sensation of the shoulder catching, clicking, stiffening, or fatiguing quickly. The pain may awaken the patient at night secondary to difficulty finding a comfortable position in which to sleep.

They may also complain of difficulty initiating shoulder abduction if the supraspinatus is involved. In addition to pain, the patient may complain of decreased active range of motion and depending on the severity of the tear, weakness.

PE   Physical examination will typically reveal painful or decreased range of motion in lifting the arm overhead or internally rotating the arm behind the back. The acromion, coracoacromial ligament, greater tuberosity, and/or the subacromial bursa may be tender to palpation. Each of the four rotator cuff muscles should be initially palpated for tenderness. There may also be associated tenderness to palpation beneath the acromion or over the acromioclavicular joint. Motor strength testing of the rotator cuff muscles can reveal weakness, depending on the severity of the tear. Also, depending on the time of injury, if the patient presents shortly following an acute rotator cuff injury, pain may be perceived as weakness, rendering strength testing less reliable.

Several provocative maneuvers may be helpful. Neer's, modified Hawkins–Kennedy, and the Empty Can tests can be positive with impingement (Figures 6-1, 6-2 and 6-3). The drop arm test involves passive abduction of the patient's arm to 90 degrees with instruction to slowly adduct the arm. Patients with a complete tear will likely be unable to hold the arm against gravity and will "drop" the arm back to neutral. Full thickness tears typically are associated with significant loss of range of motion and weakness. Chronic tears may be associated with less pain; however, the weakness and loss of range of motion persist.

FIGURE 6-1. Neer's test

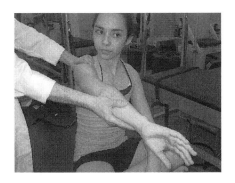

FIGURE 6-2. Modified Hawkins-Kennedy test

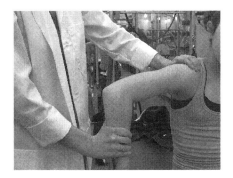

FIGURE 6-3. Empty Can test

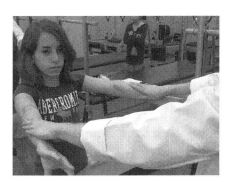

Imaging/Diagnostic Evaluation   Radiographs are helpful to demonstrate the presence or absence of a curved or hooked acromion and should include AP, lateral, and axillary views. They will also show calcific deposits within the supraspinatus tendon, if present. Radiographic changes associated with a rotator cuff tear include superior migration of the proximal humerus with reduction of the acromiohumeral distance to less than 7 mm, the presence of osteophytes and/or subacromial sclerosis [2]

MRI is very helpful to indicate the degree and extent of pathology, although false positive and false negative MRI findings are not uncommon. MRI will reveal full thickness tears and provide useful pre-operative information regarding degree of injury and any associated rotator cuff disease or soft tissue injury. Ultrasound is also useful as a dynamic technique to visualize the integrity of the rotator cuff tendons and any associated edema, hemorrhage, or calcifications.

The lidocaine impingement test, originally described by Neer, involves injection of 3–10 cc of local anesthetic, typically 1 % lidocaine or xylocaine, into the subacromial bursa. Pain relief is considered a positive test and reflective of subacromial impingement.

Treatment   Initially, **PRICE** is helpful for the acute phase of impingement and as conservative treatment of a rotator cuff tear to reduce pain, swelling, and inflammation. NSAIDs, a shoulder sling for comfort, and modalities such as ultrasound, transcutaneous electrical nerve stimulation (TENS), and cryotherapy can be helpful.

Once the pain is under control, initial physical therapy should focus on establishing proper scapulohumeral range of motion, which in dancers is paramount. Physical therapy addresses restoration of ROM and function and emphasizes gentle passive stretching of the posterior capsule. This is followed by increased active stretching, rotator cuff strengthening, scapular stabilization, and progressive resistance exercises when active pain-free range of motion is restored. Strengthening exercises of the rotator cuff and scapular stabilization exercises are important to recenter the humeral head. Also, education in proper postural alignment is essential for dancers to avoid further injury and reestablish correct scapular kinematics.

If these initial treatment measures fail, a subacromial corticosteroid injection performed in the office can help decrease inflammation and pain. It should be confirmed, however, via MRI that the patient does not have a rotator cuff tear, as corticosteroid injection can exacerbate the tear. Patients who are most likely to benefit from an intra-articular corticosteroid injection have significant subacromial inflammation that interferes with their normal activities of daily living, school or work, and is associated with severe pain or pain occurring at night.

Most patients' impingement symptoms resolve with non-operative management. Non-operative treatment of rotator cuff tears is generally effective in over 60% of patients. However, if symptoms of impingement become chronic for more than 6–12 months or in patients with rotator cuff changes on MRI, large subacromial spurs, full unrestricted PROM, and prior positive response to subacromial space lidocaine injection [3], surgical options should be considered. For recalcitrant impingement, glenohumeral arthroscopy, and open surgical decompression of the subacromial space are available therapeutic options. Glenohumeral arthroscopy is also diagnostic in cases of failed non-operative therapy to identify any associated labral, articular, or muscular pathology.

In the case of a rotator cuff tear in an elite dancer in which lifting the shoulder overhead is important and especially for symptoms persisting longer than 3 months, surgical intervention should also be considered. Research has shown that over time, the size of the rotator cuff tear progresses. If a small partial thickness rotator cuff tear on the articular surface without subacromial impingement is noted on diagnostic arthroscopy, glenohumeral debridement of the tear is recommended if the tear is less than 50% of the rotator cuff thickness [3]. If associated subacromial impingement is noted, subacromial decompression is recommended. Today, arthroscopic rotator cuff repair has generally replaced open or mini-open rotator cuff repairs and is recommended for greater than 50% partial thickness or full thickness rotator cuff tears.

Patients should be advised that 6–12 months of post-operative rehabilitation will likely be necessary prior to return to full dance activity. Patients should have pain free full range of motion with more than 80% return of strength upon return to dance [4].

Case Report   A 17-year-old male gymnast and volleyball server presents to your office complaining of the sensation of his shoulder slipping in and out of place when serving and while on the uneven bars. He has been able to voluntarily dislocate his shoulder in the past and is double jointed.

Diagnosis   Anterior glenohumeral joint instability, shoulder dislocation

Epidemiology   Anterior glenohumeral joint instability is more common than posterior instability in younger dancers and occurs with a higher recurrence rate.

Pathophysiology   The glenohumeral joint is a ball and socket joint that moves in conjunction with the scapulothoracic joint in a glenohumeral rhythm to allow abduction of the arm and rotation of the glenoid without acromial impingement. When this joint motion is balanced, a 2:1 ratio of glenohumeral to scapulothoracic motion exists. Glenohumeral joint instability is defined as translation of the humeral head on the glenoid fossa with incomplete separation. The direction of the instability may be anterior, posterior, or multidirectional. Anterior glenohumeral instability occurs more often in younger dancers, tends to recur, and is frequently associated with abduction and external rotation of the arm. Posterior instability is usually preceded by a fall onto a flexed and adducted arm and is less common than anterior instability. Dancers are at higher risk for glenohumeral joint instability with a higher incidence of hypermobility.

A shoulder dislocation can be partial or complete. If it is partial, the humeral head has subluxed to some degree out of the glenoid socket. If it is complete, the humeral head has completely dissociated from the socket. Falling onto an extended arm is the most common inciting event, although any awkward and forced position extending the arm out of the joint may result in dislocation.

History   The patient will typically complain of performing some type of movement in which the arm was abducted and externally rotated with a resultant feeling of the shoulder slipping out of place. Dislocation is usually associated with a fall onto an extended arm or outstretched hand with subsequent pain and an "unsteady" feeling in the shoulder. The patient may also complain of associated shoulder pain, numbness, tingling, and/or a feeling of shoulder weakness secondary to fatigue. The surrounding shoulder muscles may spasm in response to the dislocation. Patients with increased ligamentous and/or capsular laxity may present more frequently with glenohumeral joint instability and are more likely to dislocate their shoulders.

PE   Several provocative maneuvers can elicit anterior glenohumeral instability. The apprehension test is performed by having the patient lie supine and placing the shoulder in 90 degrees of abduction and external rotation. The apprehension test is positive when the patient subsequently feels apprehensive and fearful that the shoulder will dislocate. The relocation test should relieve this feeling of apprehension by having the examiner apply a posteriorly directed force to the anterior aspect of the shoulder. This maneuver should resolve rather than elicit apprehension. The anterior load and shift test is positive when the humeral head can be passively, anteriorly displaced on the glenoid by the examiner.

In an acute dislocation, the patient will typically minimize active movement of the shoulder and attempted passive range of motion by the examiner will be painful. Anterior instability can be assessed with the anterior apprehension test. A positive sulcus sign reflects inferior shoulder laxity. Posterior dislocation of the shoulder results in adduction and internal rotation of the shoulder, although this is rare.

Imaging/Diagnostic Evaluation   AP, scapular Y view, and axillary lateral view radiographs are recommended to adequately visualize the glenohumeral joint and assess for the presence of dislocation. They can demonstrate presence of a **compression fracture of the posterior humeral head** following traumatic contact with the anterior glenoid. This is known as a **Hill-Sachs lesion** and reflects anterior shoulder dislocation. More severe unidirectional trauma can result in a **detachment of the anteroinferior glenohumeral ligament labral complex from the anterior glenoid rim**, known as a **Bankart lesion**. Internal and external rotation views are helpful to visualize bony detail and specifically lesions involving the lesser tuberosity of the humerus. The posterolateral aspect of the humeral head can be visualized with the Stryker-Notch view, where the patient lies supine, extends the arm overhead, flexes the elbow, and supports the head with the hand. This view is useful to visualize Hill-Sachs lesions. The West Point lateral axillary view can demonstrate fractures of the anterior glenoid and is helpful to visualize bony Bankart lesions. MRI will reveal soft tissue pathology, such as Bankart lesions, more subtle Hil-Sachs deformities, and associated pathology, e. g. rotator cuff tears.

Treatment   Initially, the patient may be treated with a sling for comfort and to minimize excess motion of the joint for 2–4 weeks. An individualized physical therapy program should then focus on shoulder girdle complex range of motion exercises, including Codman pendulum exercises and progress to isotonic and isokinetic strengthening. Scapular stabilization and rotator cuff strengthening are fundamental. Dancers with associated capsular laxity will likely not be able to avoid recurrent dislocations without appropriate treatment of capsular laxity. Studies have shown significantly higher rates of dislocation recurrence in younger populations than older populations and in athletes than in non-athletes [5].

Historically, surgery was typically reserved for shoulders that dislocated three times or more. Today, however, arthroscopic repair of the Bankart lesion and capsulorrhaphy is an option for patients as early as their initial dislocation, as this is a relatively minimally invasive procedure. It also yields a low incidence of post-operative shoulder stiffness, little loss of external rotation, and results in a less than 5–10% recurrence rate.

Immediately post-operatively, the arm is placed in a sling for 4–6 weeks with precautions to avoid external rotation of the arm beyond neutral. Four weeks post-operatively, active range of motion exercises begin with arm flexion, followed by internal and external rotation of the arm with 5–10 lbweights and progress to full active range of motion by 3 months. By this time, the patient should have 70% return of external rotation, followed by 100% return of range of motion and strength by 6 months following surgery.

Shoulder subluxations can usually be relocated independently by the patient. Acute anterior dislocations can be relocated by a physician with manual downward traction on the arm and reduction of the humeral head, known as the Stimson technique. Ice and anti-inflammatory medications can help reduce pain and acute inflammation in the joint. Initially, physical therapy following the reduction is essential for rotator cuff strengthening, scapular stabilization, and the prevention of future dislocations.

Dancers are notorious for hyperlaxity in their joints, and as the shoulder joint is the most mobile joint in the body, they are at increased risk for future dislocations. Dancers with associated capsular laxity will likely not be able to avoid recurrent dislocations without appropriate treatment of the laxity. Surgical options are typically reserved for Bankart lesions or instability that does not respond to the above rehabilitation options.

Case Report   A 35-year-old male modern dancer presents to your office complaining of shoulder pain and instability following a fall onto his outstretched arm after lifting his dance partner overhead and losing his balance. The pain is worse when trying to lift his arm overhead.

Diagnosis   Glenoid labrum tear

Epidemiology   Greater incidence with repetitive throwing movements or lifts. May occur following acute injury or chronically after repetitive throwing motions.

Pathophysiology   The glenoid labrum lines the glenoid fossa circumferentially and provides insertion points for the rotator cuff and biceps tendons. Typically, a glenoid labrum tear occurs as a result of trauma or repetitive overuse injury with subsequent associated pathology to the rotator cuff and/or biceps tendons. The tear may occur in a single or multiple directions through the anterior, superior, or posterior aspects of the labrum. Compared to the rest of the labrum, the superior border may be more susceptible to traumatic and degenerative lesions due to its more meniscoid attachment. A SLAP lesion describes a superior labral tear that extends in the anterior–posterior direction and involves the biceps tendon at its origin [6]. SLAP lesions have been divided into four types. Type I involves degenerative changes of the labrum. Type II includes degenerative labral changes and detachment of the superior labrum from the glenoid rim. The biceps tendon remains intact and lifts the superior portion of the labrum. Type III injuries involve displacement of the detached superior labrum fragment into the joint, known as a bucket handle tear. Type IV injuries involve a bucket handle tear with associated partial rupture of the long head of the biceps tendon. The integrity of the biceps tendon is important to assess as this muscle contributes to glenohumeral joint stability and loss of its stabilizing function results in loss of shoulder function.

History   The patient may complain of anterior shoulder pain associated with clicking, catching, locking, and/or popping, worse with overhead activities. The pain may be localized anteriorly or felt deep in the shoulder. The patient may complain of prior fall onto an outstretched arm, direct trauma to the shoulder, a specific compression or traction injury or prior repetitive overhead activities. Throwing motions may become difficult.

PE   Physical examination with provocative maneuvers can reveal labrum instability, although several tests are sensitive but not specific. Forced hyperflexion and abduction may elicit pain if a SLAP lesion is present. The load and shift test is performed by holding the humeral head and applying an anterior, then posterior force while manipulating it in the glenoid fossa over the labrum. Excess translation of the humeral head anteriorly or posteriorly reflects labrum instability and is considered a positive test. O'Brien's test is performed by standing behind the patient while he/she flexes the arm to 90 degrees and adducts it 15 degrees medially past midline. Apply an

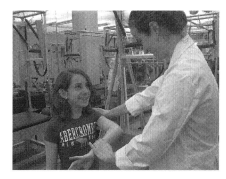

FIGURE 6-4. O'Brien's test arm pronated

inferiorly directed force on the arm while the patient internally rotates it (Figure 6-4). This will typically elicit pain in the shoulder or AC joint. Next, repeat the same exam with the forearm maximally supinated. If this reduces the pain, the test is considered positive. Deep pain is associated with labral pathology, while superficial pain is associated with AC joint pathology. If the SLAP lesion involves injury or irritation of the biceps tendon, Speed's tension test may be positive. This test is performed by resisting active shoulder flexion while the patient holds the arm in nearly complete extension with the forearm maximally supinated (Figure 6-5). Without associated impingement, Neer's, modified Hawkins–Kennedy, and Empty Can tests should be negative.

Imaging/Diagnostic Evaluation   AP, scapular Y view, and axillary lateral view radiographs are recommended to adequately visualize the glenohumeral joint and assess for the presence of dislocation. Normal radiographs are usually not valuable. MRI and especially MR arthrogram are helpful to evaluate the presence of labral tear or SLAP lesion although there is a relatively high degree of false positives and false negatives [7]

Treatment   Initially, the patient may be treated with a sling to minimize excess motion of the joint for 2–4 weeks. Relative rest with avoidance of aggravating activities should be recommended, while taking care to prevent development of a frozen shoulder. An individualized physical therapy

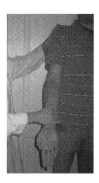

FIGURE 6-5. Speed's tension test

program should focus on shoulder girdle complex range of motion, pendulum Codman's exercises, and closed chain scapulothoracic and glenohumeral strengthening exercises.

Operative management may be required for the symptomatic patient unresponsive to conservative management. Arthroscopy will reveal the type of SLAP pathology and direct treatment. Type I lesions typically require debridement only. Type II lesions usually require debridement and reattachment of the biceps tendon to the superior glenoid rim with suture anchors. Type III lesions require excision of the bucket-handle tear and repair of any associated biceps tendon instability. Type IV lesions must be visualized to determine the degree of biceps tendon tearing. If less than 30% of the tendon is damaged, the biceps origin is left intact and only the damaged portion is resected. If more than 30% of the tendon is involved and the patient is an otherwise young, active dancer, repair of the tendon and reattachment of the labrum is performed. If the patient no longer requires maximal range of motion or high demand dance activity, especially in an older dancer, biceps tenotomy/tenodesis and labral debridement may be performed.

Case Report   A 19-year-old male modern dancer presents to your office complaining of right anterior shoulder pain that travels to his elbow and is worse when lifting his partner and when weightlifting in the gym. It occasionally bothers him at night and he feels his symptomatic shoulder tires more easily.

Diagnosis   Proximal biceps tendonitis

Epidemiology   Occurs more often as overuse than acute injury in dancers.

Pathophysiology   Biceps tendonitis as a general term is characterized by a chemical and mechanical pathology. Chemically, the long head of the biceps tendon is inflamed in the bicipital groove through which the long head courses between the greater and the lesser humerus tubercles. Mechanically, the tendon is impinged between the acromion, the head of the humerus, and the coracoclavicular ligaments. In dancers, chronic overload of the biceps tendon can lead to microscopic tears that trigger inflammation. In this example, biceps tendonitis is distinguished from tendinosis, which implies an underlying degenerative process that causes histologic changes seen as fibroplasia and scar tissue in the tendon.

History   The patient will typically complain of anterior shoulder pain over the bicipital groove that may be associated with referred pain down the biceps tendon, to the elbow or diffusely over the shoulder. The pain is usually worse with overhead activities and when loading the arm with the elbow flexed.

PE   The patient may have point tenderness to palpation over the bicipital groove. The bicipital groove can be found by first palpating the greater tubercle of the humerus and passively externally and internally rotating the shoulder. Medial to the greater tuberosity is the bicipital groove. It is important to compare shoulders as patients may have tenderness to palpation over the bicipital groove even in the asymptomatic shoulder. Several provocative tests can be helpful in diagnosing biceps tendonitis. Speed's test is performed by asking the patient to flex the shoulder against resistance with the elbow almost completely extended and forearm supinated. Pain that is reproduced at the anterior shoulder is considered a positive test. Yergason's test is performed by having the patient flex the elbow to 90 degrees while holding the elbow adducted against the body and supinating the wrist against resistance (Figure 6-6). A positive test reproduces the pain.

Imaging/Diagnostic Evaluation   No specific imaging technique can identify biceps tendonitis. It is primarily a clinical diagnosis. However, plain radiographs can demonstrate degenerative articular changes or calcifications in and around the tendon. Ultrasound can dynamically visualize the tendon in the bicipital groove with any associated edema, tears or calcifications.

FIGURE 6-6. Yergason's test

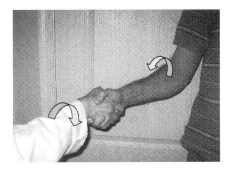

Treatment   Most patients can be treated effectively non-operatively. Initially, **PRICE** forms the mainstay of treatment. An individualized physical therapy program should then focus on progressive range of motion exercises, including Codman pendulum exercises. Modalities such as ultrasound, soft tissue release, and electrical stimulation can be helpful. Stretching and strengthening exercises should progress from isometric to concentric, eccentric, and proprioceptive exercises. If an initial course of physical therapy is inadequate in relieving the patient's pain, consider an ultrasound-guided bicipital corticosteroid–lidocaine injection. Take great care to avoid injecting directly into the tendon. Surgical intervention, usually arthroscopic, is reserved for situations where the shoulder does not respond to the above treatment options. A debridement of the biceps tendon for less than 50% thickness tear may be performed. If greater than 50% of the biceps tendon thickness is involved, a tenotomy, or in the higher demand patient, biceps tenodesis is usually required.

References

1. Dumonski M, Mazzocca AD, Rios C et al. Evaluation and management of acromioclavicular joint injuries. Am J Ortho 2004; 33(10): 526–32.
2. Sanders TG, Morrison WB, Miller MD. Imaging techniques for the evaluation of glenohumeral instability. Am J Sports Med 2000; 28(3): 414–34.
3. DeBerardino TM, Arciero RA, Taylor DC, Uhorchak JM. Prospective evaluation of arthroscopic stabilization of acute, initial anterior shoulder dislocations in young athletes. Two-to-five year follow-up. Am J Sports Med 2001; 29(5): 586–92.
4. Hawkins RJ, Kennedy JC. Impingement syndrome in athletes. Am J Sports Med 1980; 8(3): 151–58.
5. Carr KE. Musculoskeletal injuries in young athletes. Clin Fam Prac 2003; 5(2): 385–406.
6. Snyder SJ et al. SLAP Lesions of the shoulder. Arthroscopy: J Arth Rel Surg 1990; 6(4): 274–79.
7. Bencardino JT, Beltran J, Rosenberg ZS et al. Superior labrum anterior-posterior lesions: Diagnosis with MR arthrography of the shoulder. Radiology 2000; 214: 267–71.

7
Elbow, Wrist, and Hand Injuries

Case Report   A 42-year-old recreational ballroom dancer and avid golfer presents to your office complaining of elbow pain that is worse while swinging the golf club and specifically at the end of the swing before he hits the ball.

Diagnosis   Medial epicondylitis

Epidemiology: Most common cause of medial elbow pain.

Pathophysiology   Medial epicondylitis involves predominantly the forearm muscles of flexion and pronation, including the flexor carpi radialias, palmaris longus, pronator teres, and occasionally the flexor carpi ulnaris and flexor digitorum superficialis, at their origin at the humeral anterior medial epicondyle. The ulnar (medial) collateral ligament and the radial (lateral) collateral ligament stabilize the elbow. Medial epicondylitis occurs secondary to repetitive overuse most often from throwing motions with the arm overhead or serving motions as in golf and tennis. Acutely, it is typically characterized as a tendonitis and chronically as a tendinosis when the tendon fails to heal, and develops degenerative changes associated with granulated, fibrous tissue.

History   The patient may report prior acute injury, most often during a sport or dance activity that included throwing or serving. The pain may also have worsened gradually with repetition of the inciting activities. He or she will typically complain of medial epicondylar pain worse with wrist pronation and flexion. There may be associated numbness or tingling radiating into the fourth and fifth fingers if there is ulnar nerve involvement.

PE   The medial epicondyle and approximately one inch distal to the epicondyle toward the belly of the muscles are often tender with palpation. Resisted wrist flexion with the forearm pronated is typically painful (Figure 7-1). The motor, sensory, and reflex exams are useful to evaluate any associated cervical

From: *Musculoskeletal Medicine*: *Essential Dance Medicine*
By A. Bracilović, DOI 10.1007/978-1-59745-546-6_7,
© Humana Press, a part of Springer Science+Business Media, LLC 2009

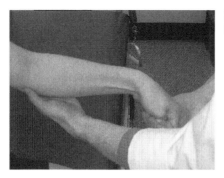

FIGURE 7-1. Resisted wrist flexion with forearm pronation.

radiculopathy and/or ulnar neuropathy. Valgus and varus testing of the collateral ligaments should be performed to assess ligament stability.

Imaging/Diagnostic Evaluation   Although no imaging techniques are diagnostic, AP and lateral elbow radiographs can evaluate any associated bony pathology. MRI will reveal integrity of the collateral ligaments and surrounding soft tissue. Nerve conduction studies and electromyography can be useful if the ulnar nerve is involved.

Treatment   Initially, **PRICE** is helpful to reduce pain and inflammation. An elbow splint that provides medial counterforce can be used to relieve pressure on the medial epicondyle and a wrist splint that keeps the wrist in neutral position can be used to relieve tension on the wrist flexors. A counterbalance brace is recommended for mild symptoms as it allows for some degree of motion while restricting full range of motion. Consider oral NSAIDs and/or a corticosteroid/lidocaine injection into the symptomatic area for pain that does not resolve. Avoid direct injection into the tendon or ulnar nerve. Physical therapy should focus on stretching and flexibility exercises initially, followed by isometric, then eccentric strengthening exercises. Modalities such as ultrasound, transcutaneous electrical nerve stimulation, and iontophoresis may be helpful. Surgical options are reserved for pain that has not responded to nonoperative management and is contraindicated in patients with any associated ligamentous instability. Surgical intervention may include epicondylar debridement or surgical pinning for an unstable elbow joint.

Case Report   A 32-year-old male trapeze artist presents to your office complaining of right elbow pain when extending his arms to lift and hold his trapeze partner in mid-air. He also has noticed the same elbow pain while playing tennis and when replacing his car tires.

Diagnosis   Lateral epicondylitis

Epidemiology   Frequent cause of lateral elbow pain.

Pathophysiology   Overuse and repetitive movements that overload the extensor and supinator tendons can lead to microtrauma and small tears of the extensor tendons, particularly the extensor carpi radialis brevis. In athletes, lateral epicondylitis is also called tennis elbow, occurring as a result of poor backhand technique, incorrect grip size, and/or excess string tension.

History   The patient typically presents with lateral elbow pain that is worse with holding and lifting objects with the arm extended. There may be associated pain and perceived weakness. The pain is usually chronic in nature, whereas acute on chronic pain is typically associated with rupture of the extensor tendons.

PE   The patient typically will have tenderness to palpation 2–5 cm distal to the lateral epicondyle over the origin of the common extensor tendon. The patient may have poor grip strength and pain while gripping objects with the arm extended. Mill's test is positive when resisted wrist extension is painful (Figure 7-2). Cozen's test is performed with the examiner placing his/her thumb over the patient's lateral epicondyle and stabilizing the elbow. The test is positive when the patient experiences pain with flexing the fingers into a fist, pronating the forearm, extending, and radially deviating the wrist against resistance (Figure 7-3). The patient may also have pain over the lateral epicondyle when the examiner places his/her thumb over the lateral epicondyle, passively extends the elbow, and forcibly flexes the wrist.

Imaging/Diagnostic Evaluation   Radiographs of the elbow are usually unremarkable, although they may reveal a lateral epicondylar spur, which

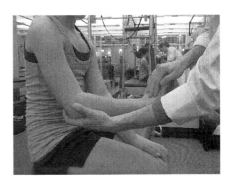

FIGURE 7-2. Mill's test.

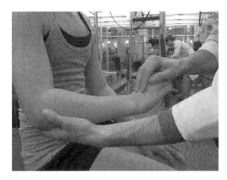

FIGURE 7-3. Cozen's test.

are usually more recalcitrant to conservative management. MRI can reveal pathology of the extensor tendons.

Treatment   PRICE is recommended as the initial course of treatment and is effective for the majority of patients. NSAIDs can be helpful in the acute phase to reduce pain and inflammation. Physical therapy should initially involve exercises to restore pain-free range of motion, improve flexibility, and progress to strengthening exercises. Use of a tennis elbow brace may also be helpful. For dancers, it is important to improve any errors in lifting technique involving use of the affected extensor tendons. If the above options fail, consider a local corticosteroid injection with care not to inject directly into a tendon. After 6 months, surgery may be considered. Surgical options include debridement of the degenerative portion of the extensor carpi radialis tendon and any associated lateral epicondylar spur.

Case Report   A 25-year-old modern dancer who works as a secretary presents to your office complaining of bilateral hand numbness, right worse than left, which has been progressively worsening. When she wakes up in the morning, she finds she often has to shake her hands to get rid of the "tingly" feeling. She types frequently at a computer during the day.

Diagnosis   Carpal tunnel syndrome

Epidemiology   Most common compressive neuropathy in athletes.

Pathophysiology   Carpal tunnel syndrome describes a median nerve mononeuropathy. The median nerve passes through the carpal tunnel at the wrist. The carpal tunnel is bordered by the transverse carpal ligament superiorly, the carpal bones inferiorly, and contains the flexor pollicis longus tendon, the four flexor digitorum profundus tendons and four flexor digitorum superficialis tendons, as well as the median nerve. Carpal tunnel syndrome can occur as a result of several mechanisms of injury that cause compression of the carpal tunnel, including arthritis, a wrist fracture, or pregnancy. Most often, the pathophysiology of carpal tunnel syndrome involves demyelination and when severe, axonal loss.

Three categories of carpal tunnel syndrome have been described, depending on the severity of symptoms. Each stage also includes specific electrodiagnostic findings. Mild carpal tunnel syndrome is characterized by paresthesias, numbness, or dysesthesias in the first three digits and may include the lateral aspect of the fourth digit. Electrodiagnostic findings consistent with mild carpal tunnel syndrome include prolonged sensory nerve action potential (SNAP) latencies and normal compound motor action potential (CMAP) amplitudes. Electromyogram (EMG) in mild carpal tunnel syndrome is typically normal. Moderate carpal tunnel syndrome is characterized by sensory symptoms along the median nerve distribution, involving both the hand and arm proximally. This stage is also characterized by impairment of fine motor coordination.

Electrodiagnostic findings consistent with moderate carpal tunnel syndrome include prolonged SNAP latencies, decreased SNAP amplitudes, and prolonged CMAP latencies. EMG in moderate carpal tunnel syndrome is also typically normal. Severe carpal tunnel syndrome is characterized by significant sensory loss along the medial nerve distribution as well as muscular atrophy of the thenar eminence. Electrodiagnostic findings consistent with severe carpal tunnel syndrome include absent SNAP amplitudes and decreased CMAP amplitudes. EMG in severe carpal tunnel syndrome typically shows abnormal activity reflective of median nerve compression.

History   The patient will typically present initially complaining of hand numbness, tingling, paresthesias in the affected hand. Most often, the symptoms include pain and paresthesias in the first three digits and the lateral aspect of the fourth finger. However, secondary to autonomic nerve fiber involvement from the median nerve, the patient's symptoms may be felt in the whole hand. The pain may be worse at night and/or progress to the arm and shoulder. It typically improves with "shaking" or "flicking" the hands upon waking in the morning. The patient may also complain of frequently dropping objects, losing grip and feeling that the hand is swollen, tight or heavy. They may have difficulty turning doorknobs or twisting objects open or closed. As symptoms progress from mild to moderate, the patient may present with decreased sensation and weakness in the hand along the distribution of the median nerve. With severe symptoms, the patient can complain of significant sensory and motor loss.

PE   Depending on the severity of symptoms, the patient's physical examination findings will likely differ. The patient may have decreased sensation to pinprick over the palmar three digits and radial half of the fourth digit. When severe, muscle weakness and/or atrophy of the median nerve innervated first and second lumbricals, opponens pollicis, abductor pollicis brevis, and/or flexor pollicis brevis may be present. Although none are pathognomonic, several provocative tests for carpal tunnel syndrome have been described. The carpal compression test is positive if paresthetic symptoms occur within 30 seconds of firm, steady pressure over the carpal tunnel (Figure 7-4). Phalen's test is positive when maintaining the wrist in 90 degrees of flexion for one minute reproduces paresthetic symptoms (Figure 7-5).Reverse Phalen's test is positive when maintaining the wrist in 90 degrees of extension reproduces the patient's paresthetic symptoms. The carpal tunnel compression test is positive when compression of the carpal tunnel for 30 seconds with the thumb reproduces

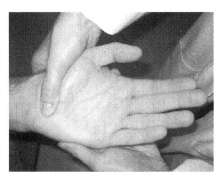

FIGURE 7-4. Carpal compression test.

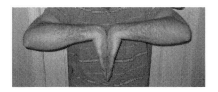

FIGURE 7-5. Phalen's test.

the patient's symptoms in the hand. When symptoms are severe, physical examination may also reveal thenar atrophy and decreased two point discrimination in the median nerve distribution of the affected hand.

Imaging/Diagnostic Evaluation   Electrodiagnostic studies including nerve conduction studies and electromyography are standard of care for the diagnosis of carpal tunnel syndrome. They are helpful to establish the degree of nerve injury and provide prognostic information. Electrodiagnostic findings can help classify the syndrome as mild, moderate, or severe. Repeat electrodiagnostic studies can be used to evaluate efficacy of treatment. No routine imaging studies are considered diagnostic for carpal tunnel syndrome. Ultrasound and MRI of the carpal tunnel can demonstrate space-occupying lesions.

Treatment   Initial treatment should include a course of physical and occupational therapy as well as a specific ergonomic evaluation of the patient's workplace. Common postural factors associated with carpal tunnel syndrome include poor sitting posture (often in front of a computer), incorrect wrist and hand placement while typing and incorrect computer monitor, chair, and table height. Patients should be instructed to avoid positions of extreme wrist flexion or extension that increase pressure on the median nerve. Custom made wrist orthoses that maintain the wrist in a neutral position can be worn at night for mild symptoms. Occupational therapy should focus on stretching techniques for the carpal tunnel as well as strengthening exercises for the hand and wrist. NSAIDs and more recently, a topical 5% lidocaine patch may be helpful to acutely reduce pain and inflammation. If a course of therapy and ergonomic rehab fail to alleviate the patient's symptoms, consider an ultrasound guided steroid injection into the carpal tunnel.

Patients with evidence of muscle atrophy, unrelieved pain, failed conservative treatment, and severe carpal tunnel syndrome as identified by electrodiagnostic studies should be considered for operative intervention. Surgery involves release of the transverse carpal ligament and can be performed as an open or endoscopic procedure. For acute carpal tunnel syndrome, an open release that provides better visualization has been recommended. The endoscopic technique typically allows faster recovery and is associated with greater risk of intra-operative nerve injury and less incisional pain. The majority of patients (>90%) have been reported to experience symptomatic relief following an endoscopic or open carpal tunnel release[1].

Case Report A 32-year-old female Broadway dancer presents to your office complaining of right hand pain after running downstage and falling forward onto her outstretched hand. She noticed swelling over the back part of her hand that is also painful to touch.

Diagnosis   Scaphoid fracture

Epidemiology Most commonly fractured bone in the wrist.

Pathophysiology The bones of the wrist, or carpal bones, consist of eight bones of which only two, the scaphoid and lunate, articulate with the radius. These bones distribute compressive forces from the hand to the forearm following a fall. The scaphoid bone itself is frequently divided into proximal, middle (waist), and distal thirds, with the middle (waist) portion most often fractured. The proximal portion is avascular and is at increased risk for necrosis following fracture, whereas the distal portion receives the greatest proportion of the blood supply. As a result, non-union is more likely to occur in the proximal and middle portions following fracture. Also, since the scaphoid bone has no ligamentous or tendinous attachments, a scaphoid fracture has higher incidence of non-union, malunion and subsequent development of arthritis [2].

Scaphoid fractures are classified as stable or unstable. Stable fractures are not displaced, are minimally comminuted, and have no associated ligamentous injury. Unstable fractures are displaced (>2 mm), significantly comminuted, and can have associated ligamentous injury.

History The patient will typically report a fall onto an outstretched hand with forced hyperextension of the wrist and pronation of the forearm. Gymnasts and modern dancers may present with a stress fracture of the scaphoid as a result of an overuse injury involving repetitive, forceful wrist extension (Figure 7-6).

PE The patient will typically have tenderness to palpation over the anatomic snuffbox (Figure 7-7), which is bordered by the scaphoid bone inferiorly, the extensor pollicis longus medially and the extensor pollicis brevis

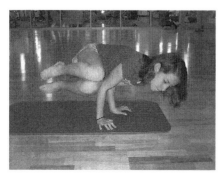

FIGURE 7-6. Wrist extension.

FIGURE 7-7. Anatomic snuffbox.

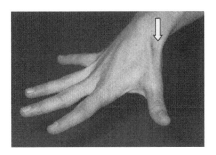

and abductor pollicis longus laterally. There may be associated swelling over the anatomic snuff box and/or wrist.

Imaging/Diagnostic Evaluation   PA, lateral, and oblique views of the wrist in ulnar deviation should be obtained. Early diagnosis and treatment of a scaphoid fracture are essential to avoid the complication of non-union. If initial radiographs are normal, CT or MRI can better define bony pathology and ligamentous injury. Radionuclide bone scanning is also useful 3–7 days following injury to identify a fracture when initial radiographs are normal.

Treatment   Stable fractures are usually treated with immobilization in a long arm thumb spica cast for 6 weeks with the wrist in neutral position, then in a short arm spica cast for 6 additional weeks. Union tends to occur by 3 months following fracture. If non-union persists as evidenced by radiograph 4 months following fracture, surgical fixation may be indicated. Following immobilization, physical therapy should include active range of motion exercises to the thumb, wrist, and forearm. The wrist should be kept neutral in a wrist and thumb splint when not in therapy.

Unstable fractures require surgical intervention with open reduction and internal fixation (ORIF). Following fluoroscopic confirmation of fixation post-operatively, the wrist should be immobilized in a short arm thumb spica cast for 6–12 weeks. About 5–10% of scaphoid fractures will result in non-union, despite appropriate treatment. Most (>90%) fractures heal appropriately if treated acutely [3]. Grafting may be required for chronic non-unions.

Physical therapy following ORIF should begin with active range of motion exercises focusing on wrist flexion, extension, pronation, supination, and mobilization of the wrist joint once the cast is removed. Elevation of the wrist following injury and surgery, if applicable, is important to minimize edema. However, it is also important to maximize mobilization of the uninjured finger, elbow, and shoulder joints to minimize disuse atrophy while allowing the bone and soft tissue heal. Strengthening exercises involving the wrist flexors and extensors should progress to resistive exercises as tolerated.

References

1. Brown RA, Gelberman RH, Seiler JG et al. Carpal tunnel release. A prospective, randomized assessment of open and endoscopic methods. J Bone Joint Surg Am 1993; 75(9): 1265–75.
2. Dias JJ, Wildin CJ, Bhowal B, Thompson JR. Should acute scaphoid fractures be fixed? A randomized controlled trial. J Bone Joint Surg Am 2005; 87(10): 2160–68.
3. Geissler WB. Carpal fractures in athletes. Clin Sports Med 2001; 20(1): 167–88.

8
Dance Glossary

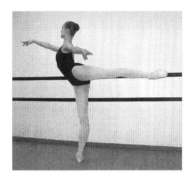

FIGURE 8-1. Arabesque.

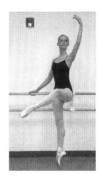

FIGURE 8-2. *Attitude en avant.*

From: *Musculoskeletal Medicine*: *Essential Dance Medicine*
By A. Bracilović, DOI 10.1007/978-1-59745-546-6_8,
© Humana Press, a part of Springer Science+Business Media, LLC 2009

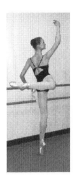

FIGURE 8-3. *Attitude derrière*, on pointe.

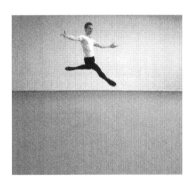

FIGURE 8-4. *Bournonville jeté.*

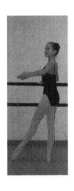

FIGURE 8-5. *Degagé.*

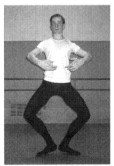

FIGURE 8-6. *Demi plié* first position heels lifted.

FIGURE 8-7. *Demi plié* first position corrected.

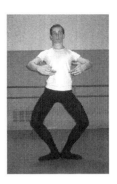

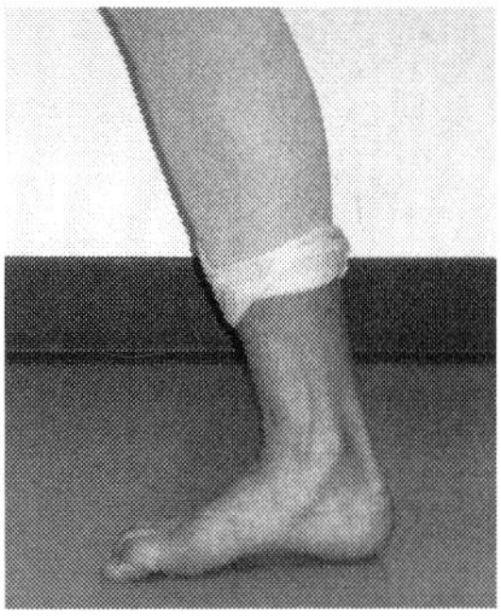

FIGURE 8-8. *Demi plié* gripping floor.

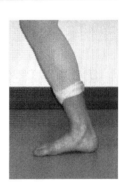

FIGURE 8-9. *Demi plié* gripping corrected.

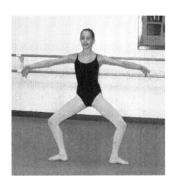

FIGURE 8-10. *Demi plié* second position.

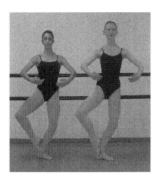

FIGURE 8-11. *Fondu coupé.*

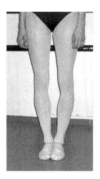

FIGURE 8-12. Genu varum.

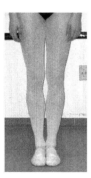

FIGURE 8-13. Genu varum corrected.

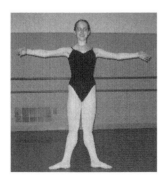

FIGURE 8-14. Genu recurvatum anterior view.

FIGURE 8-15. Genu recurvatum corrected.

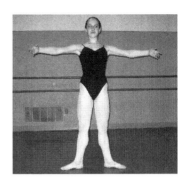

FIGURE 8-16. Genu recurvatum sagittal view.

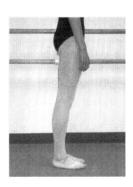

FIGURE 8-17. Genu recurvatum corrected.

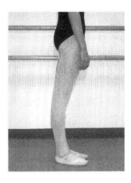

FIGURE 8-18. *Grand jeté.*

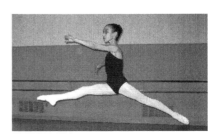

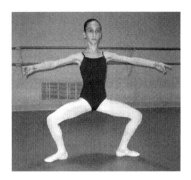

FIGURE 8-19. *Grand plié* second position.

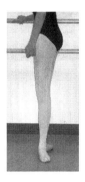

FIGURE 8-20. Overturnout first position.

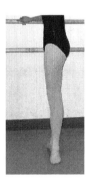

FIGURE 8-21. Overturnout corrected.

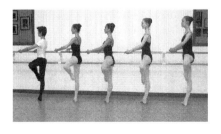

FIGURE 8-22. *Passé.*

FIGURE 8-23. *Passé développé à la seconde* hip lifted.

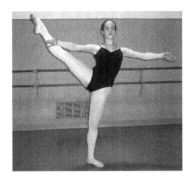

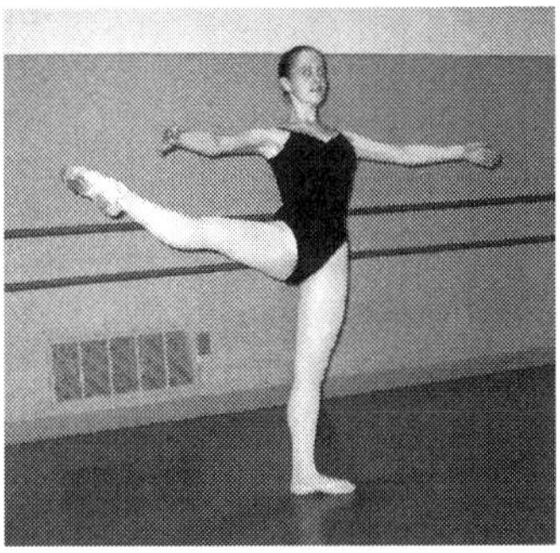

FIGURE 8-24. *Passé développé à la seconde* corrected.

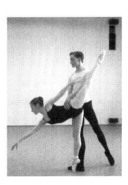

FIGURE 8-25. *Penché.*

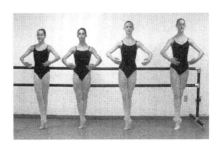

FIGURE 8-26. *Relevé sous-sus.*

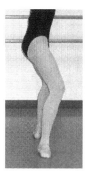

FIGURE 8-27. Second position *demi plié* overpronation.

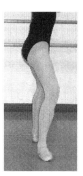

FIGURE 8-28. Second position *demi plié* oversupination.

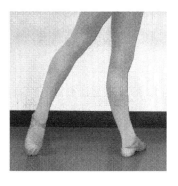

FIGURE 8-29. Tendu—sickled foot.

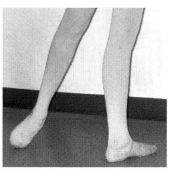

FIGURE 8-30. Tendu—winged foot.

FIGURE 8-31. Tendu corrected.

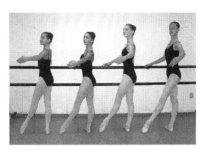

Index